Mind Estranged

My Journey from Schizophrenia and Homelessness to Recovery

a memoir by
Bethany Yeiser

All of the names of persons discussed in this book have been changed to protect their identities. The state of New Mexico is a different state, Bolivia is a different country, and the Kenyan slum of "Timunu" is a created name. All other places are factual.

Mind Estranged. Copyright © 2014 Bethany Yeiser

See bethanyyeiser.com for contact information

Printed in the United States of America

Digital Ed. ISBN 978-0-9903452-0-6
Create Space Ed. ISBN 978-0-9903452-2-0

Design by Alex Friedman, Theresa Ware and Ryan Martin

FIRST EDITION

I dedicate Mind Estranged *to my wonderful parents. I cannot thank them enough for their compassion and unconditional love. They were my most faithful and loving friends throughout my childhood, and also during and after my bout with schizophrenia. I am grateful for their many sacrifices and their refusal to give up during the darkest days of my life. I do not know if I would ever have been able to make the full recovery from schizophrenia that I have made without them.*

Table Of Contents

FOREWORD

This book is about the miraculous recovery of a highly intelligent and beautiful young lady from one of the most serious psychiatric brain disorders. Schizophrenia is a devastating mental disorder that afflicts young people in high school or college years, and usually disables them for life. The symptoms include hallucinations (hearing voices or seeing people who do not actually exist), as well as developing paranoid or bizarre beliefs that are false and unshakable. In addition, the affected young adults lose the sense of self, become apathetic and unable to initiate any action, leading to odd behavior and serious self-neglect. Their brain can no longer process information or learn new things, make decisions, or remember things. They drop out of school or college, become unable to work, deteriorate socially, and become lost in their inner psychotic world, out of touch with reality.

Although there are medications that can suppress the psychotic symptoms like hallucinations and delusions, most persons with schizophrenia remain functionally disabled for the rest of their lives because of the cognitive deficits that render them unable to continue their education, socialize, develop intimate friendships, or hold even a simple job.

The author of this book, Bethany, beat all the odds and recovered from schizophrenia, but not until the illness caused her to drop from an A to an F student, lose her college scholarship at a private university that she had achieved because of her excellent academic performance, and then become homeless on the streets of a major West Coast city for four years, with only one change of clothes, a green dress, during her last year of homelessness. Bethany was arrested and put in jail twice, but only on her third arrest did the police recognize that she was mentally ill and took her to a psychiatric ward. Her parents, who had completely lost contact with her for several years, flew immediately from Ohio to the West Coast to meet her at the hospital. The account of their gut-wrenching suffering matches that of Bethany's tragic loss of sanity and descent into homelessness.

Reading this true and gripping story of Bethany's gradual and tumultuous journey back to full mental health will open your eyes to the severe burden of schizophrenia on the affected young individuals.

It is an incredibly inspiring and hopeful story of the triumph of the human spirit. As her psychiatrist who treated her severe psychosis and hallucinations that refused to go away, helping her emerge from the hell of psychosis and returning to college to complete the requirements for a bachelor of science in molecular biology, my eyes got misty with joy as I watched her leading the procession of graduates and receiving her diploma from the university president. No one who saw Bethany during her homelessness and insanity could have ever imagined that she would return to health, pass advanced courses with As, and graduate from college with honors.

Here is a story of hope and recovery that should be read by all young people and their families who know someone with serious mental illness (25% of the U.S. population / 80 million people will have a mild, moderate or severe psychiatric disorder sometime in their lives).

Bethany is living proof that recovery is possible with good medical care, solid family support and the courage to keep fighting the tormenting voices that ordered her every move and controlled her every thought. To her great credit, she never gave up.

By writing her story, Bethany closes that painful chapter in her young life and consolidates her recovery. Sharing her personal life with others is just as therapeutic for her soul as it is inspiring to others. Her remarkable journey and the message it imparts is a source of wonderment and hope for other young persons who suffer from schizophrenia and have been written off as hopeless. But it is also a powerful message of encouragement and support for any human being facing an overwhelming challenge at some point in life. Do you know anyone who hasn't?

Henry A. Nasrallah, MD
Professor and Chairman
Department of Neurology and Psychiatry
Saint Louis University School of Medicine

INTRODUCTION

On Christmas morning 2005, I woke up on the ceramic tile floor of a public bathroom, using a shirt from my shoulder bag as a pillow. Schizophrenia turned me into a stranger, and had driven me into nearly three years of homelessness. Food was hard to come by. Underweight and hungry, I lived my homeless life within a mile of the university I attended from 1999 until 2002.

The voices began in January 2006. There was a choir of children singing, yelling, insulting me, and even complimenting me. As my sanity crumbled and faded away, I began to sleep on the grounds of a local church every night, alone.

Many years before, I lived a happy childhood filled with loving family and close friends. My teachers and professors had great expectations for me. I started college at fifteen and earned straight A's for two years. At seventeen, I served as concertmaster and first violinist of my university's community orchestra. That year, I also began working in a biochemistry laboratory. By twenty, I became the first author of a biological research article in *Proceedings of the National Academy of Sciences*, and had contributed to another paper in the *Journal of Clinical Microbiology*. My third research article in *Antimicrobial Agents and Chemotherapy* was published in 2003.

Months before I dropped out of the university, in 2002, I collaborated with university students and professionals to create a nonprofit organization to send aid to Kenya, Thailand, and other countries. I raised thousands of dollars to build a new medical clinic in Nairobi, Kenya in 2003. My future looked bright. It seemed I was a promising student that the university was destined to be proud of. But I wonder if any of their other students ever fell this far.

This is the story of how these events unfolded, how I regained my sanity, and how I came to write this memoir.

CHAPTER ONE

For a year I have slept in a churchyard surrounded by a seven-foot tall stone fence. People who notice me must know I am homeless, but I do not care.

It is winter of 2007, but I do not know the date. I sit here every day on a bench in this park for hours, thinking. Every night, I return to the churchyard to sleep. If I peer over the stone fence, I can see a dormitory with bushes and flowers in front. That is where I lived as a university sophomore. I scored A's and B's in biochemistry and molecular biology. I was going to be a medical doctor or researcher.

My small black shoulder bag was always dirty. A month ago, I threw it away, along with everything in it. Now I have no clothes, other than the green dress I am wearing, and no identification. My green dress still appears clean, but I know it is dirty. I wish I could wash it. The green dress is the only garment I own, so I do not know how I would wash it.

Years ago, wearing a dirty dress of any color would have humiliated me. But these days, my mind is a thick cloud. It is like I just found out a close friend died, and the shock never went away. I am aware that if my mind were clear, the way it used to be, I would be too embarrassed to look for leftover food in the trash, or to wear the same dirty green dress each day. But the recognition that my mind is altered makes no difference. My mind is a cloud. It prevents me from studying or working a job. I cannot concentrate.

I talk myself out of the truth that I am homeless. Homeless people look different from me. They have low cognition and appear to be dirty. They collect glass and plastic for money. I will not wander the streets gathering litter, carrying black garbage bags filled with bottles. I still have some dignity. I have never asked for money from a stranger. I have been eating thrown away food for over three years now, but I believe eating what I find is acceptable. Others hardly notice me when I look for food.

§

A few days before beginning my senior year of college, I returned from a trip to rural Africa. I was unable to make sense of what I saw there, and returned home traumatized, with a cloudy mind. I tried my best to focus on college, but shortly after my return, in the fall semester of 2002, I failed all of my courses. I became fixated on fundraising projects to assist Africa due to the extreme poverty I had seen. A year later, I raised thousands of dollars to build a small new medical clinic in Nairobi. But I was no longer capable of studying. Whenever I tried, I could not stop thinking of Africa. It constantly occupied my mind.

I dropped out of the university, but years later I still lived there. I moved around, searching for places to sleep—the libraries, the student lounges, that one restroom that had a couch. I fell asleep in other places where only students were supposed to be. I remembered the high grades I earned and the research I did, and I still felt like I was a student. But I was not a student. The university police noticed, and sent me to jail for trespassing. But there was a perk to being jailed. I was able to sleep in safety.

As I sit here in the garden, I wish I had a bed in a private, safe place where I could spend my nights, without the awful conditions in jails. Stray cats live in the churchyard, and sometimes I wish I were like them. That way, no one would accuse me of trespassing.

§

When it rains at night, and I struggle to stay dry, I want a home so badly. I wish I could work. Working any job would be a greater hell to me than the worst of the homelessness I am going through. Living in reality like a normal person makes me feel like I am in jail.

But I used to love working. I taught violin, played in orchestras, and performed for weddings. During the first two years of college, I worked full-time in two biochemistry labs, and was happy. During those years, I was on the university's meal plan. I ate whatever I wanted, whenever I wanted. I threw away leftover food without giving it a thought. Can I really be the same person?

And can homeless people speak phrases in Chinese, or have published papers in scientific research journals? Can they teach violin?

Am I even homeless? Am I crazy?

I do not know how my parents could ever understand how I have become a homeless person after so many years of school and violin practice, and after all the money they spent on my education. I have not spoken with my family in four years. I am afraid every day that they will find me in the churchyard where I sleep.

But something deep inside of me is absolutely sane, and I know I am not crazy. I often feel happy living my homeless life.

§

When I was a child, I thought that hearing voices was the craziest thing that could ever happen to a person. I am aware that I am hearing voices now, though I admit it to no one. I thought all schizophrenics were locked away somewhere forever, though I never thought of specifically where. My personality is the opposite of a schizophrenic person's. I am emotionally strong. I see just how different I am from the homeless. Would anyone ever actually group me with "them"?

I am confident I do not need to worry about my situation forever. I know the nonprofit organization my friends and I began for Africa will someday be super successful. I know that, someday, I may even be a billionaire.

Everyone will see it when it happens. The university will regret banning me from the campus when I am rich, famous, and successful. My parents will watch the news and sit in awe of my success.

§

I must have come to this park bench sometime in the morning. Now it is mid-afternoon, and I see a police officer. I am still sitting here, but I am not crazy. I am just trying to think about my childhood, and how I got here.

"Hey, are you all right?"

"Yes, sir, I just wanted some time to think. I'm fine."

"Here's my business card. Please call me at any time if you ever need help!"

"Thank you."

What a relief. He seems to be the kind of officer I grew up with, professional and caring. I do not see officers like that every day.

I still wonder if the jogger I saw yesterday with the big dog that was acting so strange around me was a drug-sniffing dog. Since I am drug and alcohol free, I will never know.

The school children have just arrived in the garden again, and I see them disembarking from a big yellow school bus. It is late afternoon, and shadows extend across the garden.

Today, as I watch the children, I am questioning why I prefer my homeless life. How did I end up here?

CHAPTER TWO

An expansive dome of blue sky and golden cornfields mark my earliest memories of rural Illinois. My dad was pastor of a 150-year-old church located between two farms, a short walk from our home.

When I was eighteen months old, my mom gave birth to my brother, who became my best playmate. I remember playing with him outside in our sandbox, and inside with toys on the carpet of our small house. My brother and I felt loved, safe, and happy. In spring, I helped mom plant seeds in our garden that touched the neighbor's cornfield. She was my best friend, even though she was so much taller than I was back then. My mother sewed all of my clothes and made matching outfits for my dolls. My parents loved living in the country.

From my earliest years, my parents worked to give my brother and me every opportunity. Our family relocated to a neighborhood in a suburb of Cleveland, Ohio when I was five. My father's new church had strikingly beautiful stained glass, including a huge stained glass cross. I can still see it now—red and blue, catching a glint of sunlight and refracting it across the pulpit.

Our new house was near a small private school I attended for grammar school and the first two years of high school. My brother and I loved taking walks with my mom and our grey puppy, Sparky.

The private school my brother and I attended was located on the grounds of a local church. I wore a plaid uniform every day and carried a red lunch box. My first grade teacher loved to travel. She gave me a pen she bought in Israel that said "I Love Israel" with "love" symbolized by a big red heart, and I kept that pen for many years. It prompted me to dream of visiting foreign countries and studying other languages. I spent ten years attending the private school.

In first grade, I began collecting coins from all over the world. I loved separating the coins by country, and eventually had a collection representing over a hundred countries. When I looked at them closely, I noticed that one coin was exceptional, since it was the only one with a hole in its middle. The coin was from Hong Kong. I used to look at the coin and dream of travelling there.

§

I was different than other kids, even in my youngest years. At school, I felt no one was quite like me and I did not "fit in" with my classmates. I often preferred talking with adults or spending time alone rather than socializing with my peers. When other kids were playing during recess, I spent time talking to my teachers, especially my fourth grade teacher.

I longed to develop closer relationships with children in my classes. When I became a teenager, my close friends became adults in their twenties from our church who welcomed me to spend time with them.

I would struggle to make friends throughout my life.

§

Our church built a new house for my family on its six acres of wooded land when I was seven. My brother and I watched with excitement and anticipation as a contractor laid the cement that would become the foundation of our house. We walked in the wooden frames that later became our rooms. Outside, we built forts out of plants and sticks and raked away weeds and shrubs to create a bike trail. My dad built us a two-story tree house.

Over the years, my brother was a wonderful playmate. He was witty, fun, and noticed everything. The two of us were very different. He was athletic, and later on, loved to snow ski, rollerblade and skateboard. In contrast, I enjoyed playing the piano and violin. While my brother could accomplish anything technically difficult, he did not love school like I did. When we were teenagers, he said the two of us were like a "photograph and a negative."

§

I began studying piano with my dad at age five, and violin at seven. My parents drove me to violin lessons every Saturday. One of my favorite childhood memories is playing violin while my dad accompanied me on the piano. We did this often. By the time I was thirteen, I practiced for several hours every day. My parents purchased a lovely violin for me, and I was accepted into the best orchestra in the area for teenagers.

From age fourteen to sixteen, I spent the summers living at a distinguished music school. There were about 150 musicians from all over the United States, and several international musicians. I finally developed close friendships with other teenagers who shared my passion for music. A Chinese girl became my pen pal. The summers were filled with fun and excellence in music as we enjoyed living on the school's ivy-covered campus filled with beautiful gardens.

Throughout my childhood, my family met many people from countries in Europe, Southeast Asia and the Middle East though our church. My parents invited them into our home, and I sat for hours listening to them describe their travels. I learned to use chopsticks at an early age and wanted to study Chinese.

As a teenager, my dad encouraged me to begin learning Biblical Greek. I began teaching myself Greek from one of his textbooks. I never progressed far with Greek, but I loved the challenge of learning a new language.

§

In high school, I planned on becoming a professional musician and was preparing to audition at music conservatories. My parents made a sacrifice to buy me a much nicer and more expensive violin, so that I could compete. I was intrigued by studying other cultures, other religions, and international politics.

In my junior year, I enrolled in a program offered through our local community college that allowed students to simultaneously earn high school and college credit. I missed my classmates from private school, but after a month, I made some friends who were serious students like me. I dove into a full-time class load at the community college, and I loved it.

When not studying, I continued to practice the violin for many hours every day, and, unfortunately, my schedule left me little time for a normal social life.

§

At the completion of my senior year, I had earned sixty-three credit hours of college. I was amazed at how the physical world could be described and understood through mathematics. I had grown to love the challenge of logical and analytical thinking in science courses. The college courses were broadening my view of academic possibilities. I toyed with the idea of becoming both a professional musician and a physicist.

I had scored high on my standardized tests. During the fall of my senior year, I received letters and brochures from over thirty American universities and colleges that were impressed by my test scores and grades. Most of my peers who were young musicians were extremely competitive. When young violinists decided to study academics instead of music, they were pleased. It was as though, by not majoring in music, student violinists had dropped out. But as I continued to receive information from universities, I considered the endless career opportunities available in academic majors.

§

On an October day in my senior year, 1998, I received a thick and colorful brochure from an excellent university decorated with faces of students of various ethnicities. I knew the school because it had a well-known music program. After thumbing through the brochure, I learned that the university was renowned for science and engineering. It quickly became my first choice school.

In spring of my senior year, my dad and I flew two thousand miles west to visit my first choice university so I could audition for the music program. We toured the campus with its fountains, ivy-covered brick buildings and stone statues. A central auditorium boasted decorative carved stone columns in rose, tan and white. The stunning campus had been created to celebrate learning. I fell in love with the university, and I was certain that I would attend, regardless of the outcome of my violin audition. I was excited about my future.

After my return to Ohio, I found out I had been turned down by the university's music program. But I announced to my parents that I intended to attend the university anyway, and that I would change my major to science. My parents were surprised by the change, but recognized my decision was sensible. They saw all of the new possibilities my decisions brought. I imagined myself as a scientist.

§

The summer after my senior year of high school, a family friend arranged a special opportunity for me to do laboratory research with a biochemistry professor at a university in downtown Cleveland. From my first day in the research laboratory, a technician taught me techniques for replicating DNA and identifying proteins. I mastered other laboratory skills, and my experiments shed light on enzymes that destroyed antibiotics, causing patients to become resistant to medication. Collecting data was exhilarating, and it felt meaningful.

During the summer, I met frequently with a geneticist whose family lived in our neighborhood, and he explained how some of the DNA techniques I was using worked. He gave me a biochemistry textbook, and through independent study, I deepened my knowledge of basic biochemistry. At the end of the summer, I knew I wanted to study HIV and AIDS, and I made the decision to major in molecular biology.

§

A large scholarship, financial aid, and my parents' financial support made it possible for me to attend my first choice university out west.

Unfortunately, entering the university was one of the most difficult times of my life. I expected that living in the honors dormitory would be like going to summer violin school again, but when I moved into the dormitory, I was shocked at the immaturity of the students. The average age at the community college I had attended full-time for two years was twenty-seven. I had not been treated like a child since tenth grade, before attending the community college. I found life in the dormitory humiliating.

My first classes at the university were disappointing. A humanities professor gave me a cold, apathetic look when I tried to ask her a question. I went to her office hours to give her another chance, but she seemed as uninterested in me as she had been in class. I had always attended professors' office hours at the community college to ask lots of questions and to get to know the professors, and I was devastated by her lack of enthusiasm about teaching. I dropped her class, my first at the university, hoping to find more dedicated professors.

My freshman biology class had hundreds of students. After spending the summer studying biochemistry on my own, there was little to learn, and I was bored. But when I visited the professor, I found he was interested in me and in the other students. He was brilliant.

My third class, on the recent history of Southeast Asia, was a delightful surprise. I was fascinated by the texts for the class. I studied hard in the ivy-covered university libraries, sitting near other serious students, loving every minute.

My first semester classes at the university in the fall of 1999 included Asian history, biology and organic chemistry. Though my initiation into the university had been rocky, I loved the academic challenge I found there.

§

From the day I arrived at the university, I wanted to do research again, and I could not wait. I found a professor who was impressed by my research from Cleveland. He welcomed me to volunteer even before classes began. In hindsight, it was probably unwise to take on this work during my first semester, but I was eager to seize the opportunity.

My first week at the university, I also auditioned for the university community orchestra and was chosen to be concertmaster. During our December performance, I would have the honor of tuning and leading the orchestra.

As fall of 1999 flew by, I spent all of my free time studying DNA replication on my own. After countless hours of independent research, I had a solid understanding of DNA replication in bacteria, humans, and in viruses like HIV, though this left me with no time for developing friendships.

I scored A's in all my classes, except organic chemistry, in which I earned a B. Getting B's was unusual for me, and I was disappointed.

§

After my first semester at the university, I returned to Ohio to spend Christmas of 1999 with my family. My parents expressed concern about the extensive amount of time I spent in the laboratory, which prevented me from having a normal social life. The laboratory was keeping me from achieving straight A's. We did not agree with each other as much as we had in previous years.

During Christmas break, I was persistently unhappy. I could think of nothing but school and my laboratory work, and I could not tolerate taking a break. On Christmas Day, I enjoyed opening presents with my family, but I left the celebration to write an email about DNA to my university research supervisor. My professor wrote me a long email in return, answering my question and encouraging me to keep reading. I received it on Christmas Day in the evening.

The best part of the winter break was when my family celebrated the long-awaited New Year's Eve of 2000, Y2K. Our house was packed with friends I had known my whole life. We had games, fireworks, and all sorts of snacks and desserts. At midnight, we watched the ball drop in New York on television as we sang "Auld Lang Syne." I finally felt like myself, enjoying old friends and family as I had in the past. But as soon as New Year's Eve was over, I became unhappy again. I had little desire to be with old friends. All I wanted was to go back out west and continue working in the laboratory.

§

Spring semester of 2000, my freshman year, I began a new project in the laboratory. The project required knowledge of the DNA replication processes I had studied independently. A professor taught me a laboratory procedure that we used to learn how bacterial DNA changes with time. I became obsessed with my research, often working in the laboratory until three o'clock in the morning or later. My dormitory was a ten-minute walk from the laboratory, and I felt safe walking back at night. In hindsight, I should have called for university escorts.

Accumulating data soon took over my coursework, and I spent little time studying. I did not have enough time that spring to stay in the orchestra, so I resigned as concertmaster. I was left with no close friends.

But after a few months, my discovery enabled my professor and me to better understand how bacterial DNA changes. It proved to be relevant and significant in the field. I was asked to publically present the findings from my months of research, and I invited every professor I knew in the department to see my presentation.

When all of my semester grades dropped, I did not care.

CHAPTER THREE

At the university, I was almost always alone. I preferred to eat by myself in the cafeteria and quickly run back to the lab. There were countless opportunities for undergraduates to see the city's downtown and go on field trips, but I never had time.

I did not really know anyone in my honors dormitory, apart from my roommate. She was brilliant with computers, and kept an exciting social life as a member of the university band. Sometimes she questioned me about why I did nothing but work and study, but we rarely talked. When Thanksgiving break came, and we were both stuck in the dormitory, we went to Denny's to have Thanksgiving dinner together. It is one of my only memories of her.

I was the only undergraduate doing research in the lab. I knew some of the doctoral students and post-docs a little, but they were also busy.

§

Despite not having a social life, I was set on attending church services every Sunday, as I had always done. I enjoyed church during my childhood.

Initially, I risked feeling awkward and out of place by visiting new churches, but when I found a church that had many international students and Americans who traveled the world, I decided to attend regularly. I hoped to make interesting friends and hear about their experiences abroad. On Sundays, I got up early to visit the laboratory before walking to the church service.

§

When summer of 2000 arrived, I moved into a different university dormitory. A student I had met through church became my roommate.

My roommate was extremely intelligent and kept a well-balanced social life. We spent time together eating ice cream, swimming, and walking the university track under the lights late at night. Since I rarely had close friends, spending free time with my new roommate that summer was special for me. I occasionally joined her and her friends on outings, and she introduced me to her family. She had grown up in Bolivia, was bilingual, and told me all about her travels.

During the summer, a university in the east delayed sending my professor some strains of bacteria, and experiments were postponed for many weeks. I wanted to work more than sixty hours in the lab every week, and the delay caused me to become even unhappier than I had been during my Christmas break. But I began to realize I was being absurd for wanting to work sixty hours a week when I should have been enjoying my free time.

At that time, I had no idea just how much more restless I would soon become.

When summer of 2000 was nearing its end, my mom visited me at the university, and we renewed our friendship. We had a lovely time together walking the campus. I showed her the laboratory. My mom helped me move into a different university apartment for the next school year.

§

During the fall of my sophomore year, 2000, I wanted to put my greatest focus into my classes as I had done in high school. I was still in the laboratory, but there was little to do. I tried to study for my courses while at the laboratory.

That fall, I began losing my ability to focus on schoolwork, and this was a new problem for me. I was becoming unable to read for more than a half hour at a time. I opened textbooks and always attended lectures, but I was shocked to see I could no longer concentrate like I used to be able to. Even with my additional free time, I found myself getting B's rather than A's in classes that would have been easy for me years prior.

I petitioned for several of my community college credits to be transferred to the university during the fall semester. I had been told by an admissions representative that the transfer would go through with no problem, but it did not.

§

The professor who supervised my research project in

Cleveland in 1999 kept in touch with me after I left for the university. He believed in me. He had no idea that my mind was deteriorating, as it was not yet obvious to anyone.

That fall, 2000, the professor invited me to attend the Interscience Conference on Antimicrobial Agents and Chemotherapy (ICAAC) in Toronto. I was scheduled to present a poster displaying the research I did in his laboratory. The ICAAC was held in late September.

Attending the ICAAC was an unforgettable professional experience. I spoke about my poster with many scientists. I was included with a group of medical doctors in activities, and was treated like a professional. We drove together to Toronto from Cleveland, and then back to Cleveland, as we talked for hours about research in medicine. We discussed my dreams of becoming a research scientist.

When the conference ended, I had every reason to work hard in my university classes and do my best to achieve my dreams. But something inside of me had changed. I told myself that my problem was that most of my dual high school and college credits had not transferred, and I was angry that I could not graduate early as I planned to. But had I been in my right mind, I would have taken extra classes in mathematics, science and foreign languages. I used to love these subjects.

When the fall semester of my sophomore year came to an end, and I scored all B's in my easier classes, I felt disgusted with myself.

CHAPTER FOUR

Christmas of 2000 was my last Christmas in the house where I grew up. My parents planned to move to Cincinnati where my dad would become pastor of a new church. Even though home was a place I had always loved dearly, I felt restless again over the break.

When I returned to the university to begin the spring semester of 2001, the second semester of my sophomore year, I completely stopped spending time in the laboratory. That spring, I took my hardest classes and scored my best grades. Somehow, I managed A's in advanced biochemistry, engineering physics, and a Spanish class. I took differential equations, a notoriously difficult class, and earned a B. I was not quite myself, but I loved my studies.

I began attending social events at my church, but, as always, it was difficult for me to make friends. I eventually got to know more people there, including many international students.

In retrospect, I realize I always had an easier time fitting in with people who did not fit in well themselves, sometimes including international students. I was intrigued by the stories I heard about international friends' experiences abroad. Sometimes, through listening to friends' stories, I felt like I was entering a new world.

One of the families from my church sought to draw me into their social circle and invited me to attend various church functions. With their encouragement, I decided to become more involved in the church. I knew my life was out of balance, that I had very few friends, and that I was unable to study as effectively as I had in high school. I hoped attending church would help me have a more balanced life and concentrate more effectively.

I began attending a church counseling program where I watched church staff interact with poor people in the city, talking with them through difficult times they were having. The counseling program enabled me to meet underprivileged individuals in the city.

§

One Sunday morning at church, I met a young Caucasian woman who had just returned from a year-long stay in Africa. After returning from Africa, she took time to debrief with a family from my church and to discuss the "poorest of the poor" she had interacted with in Africa. Friends told me she was an unusual and special person. Her name was Susan.

When I met her for the first time, I saw Susan had a wisdom that seemed quite unlike that of any person I had ever met. Friends and acquaintances of all ages sought her advice on many topics though she was only in her mid-twenties. She appeared confident, beautiful and poised. My friends were convinced that her work in Africa would have a great and far-reaching impact. It was what I wanted for myself. I became jealous of her.

I tried to figure out exactly what it was that made Susan unique. I wondered if living in poverty was the source of her unusual and broadened world perspective.

I had a brief conversation with Susan before she returned to her home in the northeastern United States. When pressed, she spoke of a suffering most Americans have never encountered. She seemed to carry a heavy burden. It was as though she carried an emotional scar in her heart.

After Susan left, I could not stop thinking about her, and my thoughts became unrealistic. I began to see her as one of the best people on earth, and barely human. I was becoming delusional. This was the first time I had ever been delusional.

I wanted to experience whatever it was that made Susan unique. I wondered if living in Africa and witnessing extreme poverty would make me more like her, or at least more able to understand her. As I thought about Susan, all the plans I had made for my life became less important to me. What I wanted most in my life was to visit Africa.

§

During my sophomore year, many of my friends were applying and being accepted to medical schools. Just like in high school with the other violinists, I wanted to compete with the premedical students. I felt extra pressure to attend medical school. The summer of 2001, following my sophomore year, I planned to take the Medical College Admissions Test (MCAT). I planned to apply to medical schools during the next summer, after my junior year, 2002.

I mentioned my desire to visit Africa to many people at my church. A pastor challenged me to become a medical doctor in order to help people in impoverished countries. Others expressed how effective I could be with higher education, going to Africa later on as a doctor or researcher, perhaps one specializing in HIV.

Academically, it seemed that a trip to Africa during my undergraduate years would be a valuable experience that could help me achieve my professional goals. Against the advice of some, I was determined to go as soon as possible.

§

That summer, 2001, I applied to become a teacher for an SAT preparation course through a company and was hired and trained to teach. As I studied for the MCAT during the summer, I had a lot of extra time, but I found myself unable to work for the company. It seemed too boring for me, and a waste of time. I would have loved the job a year before, but I could no longer focus on working. It was the same kind of struggle I had with my courses.

Somehow, at the end of the summer, I took the MCAT and scored well.

CHAPTER FIVE

Fall semester of 2001 marked my junior year at the university. I found myself producing poor grades again. I had an even more reduced ability to maintain my concentration than during my sophomore year. Friends I studied with were perplexed at how restless I was.

My church decided to send a group of students to China over Christmas break of my junior year. I was invited to join the international trip. It was paid for in full by humanitarian donors who felt the trip was a valuable experience for students.

The purpose of the China trip was to develop friendships with farmers living deep in the southwestern mountains. There were additional plans to revisit these people in the future and help them improve their farming methods. The prospect of visiting China excited me. In October of 2001, I obtained my first passport and a visa to visit China. My childhood dream of visiting the ancient country was coming true.

§

Even while I was preparing to leave for China, Susan was still living in my mind. My impression of her was tremendously unrealistic, but it did not diminish with time. Instead, it grew.

During the fall of 2001, I would score some of the lowest grades I ever had in my life, including C's. I lied to myself that my poor grades were not because of my inability to study, but because I was busy preparing to travel. I told myself the trip was more important. My mind was deteriorating further, but I could not recognize it was happening. I thought of how I used to excel in school, and I believed I still could if I really tried.

§

I flew to my parents' new home in Cincinnati to spend a few days there over Christmas before flying back to the university and leaving for China. Like previous Christmases, I felt uncomfortable with my family. I was irritable and unhappy. I did not care about the drop in my grades in classes that I would have loved years before. I was anxious every minute to leave for China, and my mind was always jumping ahead to the next activity.

My personality was beginning to change. My parents were at a loss to understand the change, and perplexed. Our conversations became strained.

As I obsessed over my plans to visit Africa as soon as possible, I never thought of my musical experiences, my former love of learning, the people in my life who I cared about, or the love I once had for my family. I needed to know what Susan had encountered in Africa that made her so special. Nothing else mattered.

§

I returned to the West Coast with one day to prepare for the trip. Flying so far away was intimidating, but the other women all had experience traveling internationally. They were also all five years older than I was. At first, I felt safe traveling with them, but later on, I felt I was smarter than them, and that I should be our group leader.

§

It was a dark, foggy night when we arrived in Beijing. On our one-night layover there, before flying south, we walked the streets of the capital and visited Tiananmen Square. The next day, we flew to a busy city in Southern China where I encountered a poor woman who approached me, grabbed my arm, and would not let me go free until I gave her money. I was frightened by the experience, but I realized the woman's desperation in her poverty.

We boarded a bus to travel far into the mountains, and after a long distance, we exited off a Chinese highway. After we traveled on narrow, rocky dirt roads, we arrived at a rural area filled with Chinese farming communities. I saw small mud huts and drainage ditches on both sides of a narrow dirt road.

§

I continued to have difficulty focusing on the present and was continually thinking about my future plan to visit Africa, even while in southern China. I was overwhelmed by the poverty in China. I told my travel companions how much I appreciated the honor of getting to see poor villages as though I were confused. It was somehow as though I considered visiting the poor to be a mark of prestige.

During the trip we began learning a few Chinese phrases, such as "What is your name?" and "How much does it cost?" I was overly eager to interact with people despite my heavy accent, and the other young women noticed it.

§

As the days passed, we visited several more farming communities. We met a poor woman who invited us into her hut and offered us a snack of seeds and nuts. We interacted with kind leaders of villages, and we found Chinese restaurant owners delighted to welcome American women. One night, while camping on a mountain, I looked up at the sky and saw it was brilliant with the Milky Way and other stars. It looked like the cover of a *National Geographic* magazine. I still continued to think of Susan, and of Africa.

§

On our return trip to America, we spent another night in Beijing. That night, I saw a Chinese woman with a baby on a sidewalk underneath a huge bridge. They were barely sheltered from the cold rain. I was horrified at the sight, and gave her five American dollars, a small fortune to her. I was devastated that I could not do more for the baby. I was shattered by the poverty I witnessed everywhere in China. To comfort myself, I rationalized that the people in poverty were happy. I told myself they still could have great lives like wealthy Americans.

I never talked through my thoughts and feelings with others who had international experience when I returned to America. This was a mistake.

§

I returned from China just as the spring semester of my junior year was beginning. When I arrived back at my apartment, I received an email notifying me that my two research projects—one from the laboratories in Cleveland, and the other from the university—had both been submitted for publication. I believed God was blessing me because I tried to help the poor.

CHAPTER SIX

I resolved I would go to Africa during the summer after my junior year, in 2002. I emailed Susan to ask her if she knew where I could live and volunteer in Nairobi.

It took a while to hear back from Susan, but after several days, she finally responded. In an email, she warned me that going to Africa to serve the poor was a painful road to take. She said it was a much more difficult journey than I might imagine, and she strongly challenged me to rethink my plans.

Susan's advice for me to reconsider my trip was unexpected, and it surprised me. But throughout my whole life, difficult challenges have always been exciting for me. I was certain I still wanted to go.

§

Susan explained that the people she knew in Nairobi usually checked their email only once a week. It took a month, but I finally received an email from a medical doctor who lived in Nairobi and knew Susan. He directed several clinics staffed by Kenyan medical professionals. There was a Kenyan woman named Naomi who lived walking distance from one of the clinics, in a certain slum. Naomi was in her late twenties and had put up destitute teenage girls at her small house for a few years. Some of the girls volunteered regularly at the clinic. In an email, Naomi invited me to rent from her while I volunteered.

When my plans to spend the summer living in Nairobi with Naomi were finalized, I was excited and relieved. My dream of visiting Africa was coming true. But I knew that Susan had spent significant time in West Africa as well as the East. For months, I tried to make contacts in West Africa, but had no success.

In the spring of 2002, I contacted the church in Cleveland where my father had been the pastor, and where I had attended every week from when I was five years old until I left for college. I asked if they might consider funding my trip to Africa. I expected I would find great support for my trip there.

Friends from my Cleveland church welcomed news of my

upcoming trip to Africa. They flew me to Ohio to visit them for a weekend, and while I was there, the church gave me a check to cover all of my expenses for flying to Africa and living there. They prayed with me. They seemed proud of the decision I was making, and they wanted to hear about my trip over email while I lived in Africa and again when I returned to America.

§

As I prepared to go to Africa, my vulnerable mind was changing. That spring, 2002, I took some of the easiest classes at the university, including general education classes, but did mediocre work. It was frustrating to take extra classes since many of the college courses I had taken in high school did not transfer. While my credits did not transfer, the university encouraged their own students to take classes for dual high school and college credit. At one point, I explained my academic situation to an older friend at the university. He told me plainly that if I was so unhappy and felt so cheated, I should transfer to another university immediately. But I was too close to graduating, and I had already transferred from the community college.

With time, I had developed an obsession with becoming like Susan that was so strong, I could think of almost nothing else. When I tried to study, my thoughts went back to my plans to visit Africa. While I prepared to visit Africa, I scored C's.

§

In addition to losing my love of learning, in 2002, I acquired a few strange habits. I walked up to an attic above the dormitory, where I lived my freshman year, and spent time there thinking or eating my lunch. It was a secluded place, and I doubt if any of the other students ever went there at all. I wanted to be in a place where no one ever went, and be totally alone at times when people socialize, such as at lunch.

I found another secluded spot in the university library at the bottom of a staircase where no one ever seemed to go. My freshman year, I sat at tables and desks and blended in with the other students as one of them. But during my third year at the university, I wanted to be so alone that no one would ever think of coming where I was. I was not paranoid, but my behavior was changing. I now see my behavior was becoming strange.

§

Prior to leaving for Africa, one of my friends in the university's master of music program recognized I was a good enough violinist to work as a professional musician. She recommended I join in playing for companies that paid string players well. She drove us to recording studios. It was fun to be paid well for something I loved doing. It was one of my only lifelines to the way my life used to be.

§

My brother and I had our university spring breaks the same week that year, 2002, two months before I left for Africa. He drove in from his university in North Dakota with some of his friends to visit me for the week. We went to nice dinners, talked, and drove all around the city. While I was with him, I felt like myself again. We had fun. I believe my brother did not notice any change in me at that time.

The week before I left for Nairobi, in early June of 2002, my parents visited me for several days. They wanted to see the university and take me on long drives into the lovely surrounding area and the desert, and to quiet places where we could talk, discussing my life and dreams. I had always loved telling them about my favorite classes and about what I was learning. I used to talk on and on about my research experiences and opportunities to play my violin. But that week, I talked little with them about my classes since my grades had dropped. I was certain they would not understand. I believed they would be proud of me after I returned from Africa. I was going to change the world through my trip.

I had begun fasting about once a week or more before going to Africa. Though I had known people at the church who fasted occasionally, I was doing it too often, and it became an unhealthy habit. When my parents visited me, they did not understand why I wanted to fast. One day, when they were happy to see me, they took me to a restaurant, and I would not eat.

I was embarrassed by the change in myself, and I was cold to my parents for no reason other than because my mind was deteriorating. Prior to leaving for Africa, something was wrong with me, and I was truly not myself.

CHAPTER SEVEN

I went to Africa to see the HIV epidemic firsthand and to volunteer in a small medical clinic. I wanted to help people in dire need of medical attention. I hoped to understand the lives and culture of the people. I wanted to become like Susan.

I transferred to Nairobi through a small airport packed with black Africans in Addis Ababa, Ethiopia. When some men saw I was alone, they began freely and deliberately stepping in front of me, and one of them was patting me on the back. It seemed my trip to Africa was off to a bad start.

I located a well-dressed and beautiful black African woman with a gold chain and kind face. She had observed my awkward situation and welcomed me to sit beside her. She was not Ethiopian, but Kenyan, and spoke English. As she began telling me about her life, she explained that she adopted several orphaned Kenyan children over many years. The woman had traveled to a conference in Ethiopia to gain financial support for her work with orphans in Nairobi.

When I noticed her gold chain, she seemed embarrassed. She tried to explain that her gold was appropriate when raising money, but that she would not be wearing it at home.

We discovered that we were both taking the same flight into Nairobi, and that she was acquainted with my Nairobi host, Naomi. I was grateful to have a new Kenyan friend, and a kind traveling companion.

§

Most Caucasians entering Kenya had great interest in its wildlife, landscapes and safaris, but I had tunnel vision to help the poor, something many of my new Kenyan friends would not understand.

After I exited Kenyan customs and found my two suitcases, I met Naomi. She wore a black suit coat lined with grassy green colored trimming and looked respectable and lovely. She was serious and quiet. I noticed she had a gravity and wisdom about her that reminded me of Susan.

Though Naomi had grown up in poverty, she was smart, and had attended high school and college on full scholarships. Later in the summer, Naomi would tell me about why she made the decision to house desperately poor teenage girls and to raise money to help them rather than finding a good-paying Nairobi job. I would find she was like Mother Teresa, sacrificial and caring.

Some of the girls I would be staying with came to meet me at the airport. They were shy, and spoke poor English, but they could communicate. They were friendly. I thought some of them were strikingly beautiful, slender and strong. Their ages ranged from about twelve to eighteen.

§

After leaving the Nairobi airport, a missionary from Germany who did not speak English drove me, Naomi and the girls through the crowded and dirty downtown to the open wilderness, and then finally to the slum. As we drove, I saw the inner city was overrun with cheap markets packed with Kenyan people. There were tables loaded with food, clothing and jewelry. I saw a little boy who was about thirteen, and Naomi recognized him as a young gang member and dangerous. It was confusing and heartbreaking to see young children who were already hardened criminals. They were everywhere.

After we drove out of the dirty, congested part of downtown Nairobi, we came to a huge highway road that penetrated a wide, empty landscape with nothing but tall grass stretching in all directions. There was a clear, bright blue sky.

It was evening when I was driven to the small concrete house where I would live with its huge gate and padlock doors. Naomi said the slum was called Lakisama. In America, I had never seen an area with so much security on houses. The need for all of the padlocks made me feel unsafe. I was right to think it was dangerous.

§

My first morning in Africa I drank tea with the girls, and we prepared to walk through Lakisama. Outside their concrete, padlocked home, I saw children running along a dirt road without shoes. Chickens ran in the paths with the children. There was a ravine nearby with garbage spilled along it, at least ten feet deep and hundreds of feet long. A small bridge extended over the ravine. I saw people everywhere, cheap dwellings with sheet metal roofs and dirt roads disappearing over hills.

Despite their poverty, the children appeared to be having fun as they played on the slum's dirt paths. Wherever I went, children yelled out to me "Mzungu! Mzungu!" the Swahili word for "white person." They were curious to see me.

§

A few days after my arrival, some of my Kenyan friends, including two men, walked with me for fifteen minutes to reach the local medical clinic. The clinic building's waiting room was about forty by forty feet with several wooden benches, and it was packed with sick people. That day, I watched small children receive Meningitis vaccinations. Though I was happy to know the children would be immune to the disease, it was horrible to watch them all breaking into tears.

I was careful to stay with the Kenyan girls and young men who traveled to the clinic with me. I could never be alone there, even for a few minutes, without big, tall men who were strangers bothering me.

§

A few days after my arrival in Africa, when I was planning to visit the clinic, tribal warfare erupted near the girl's home. I took Naomi's suggestion and went to visit other parts of Nairobi with the girls. We visited a rural area called Dandora that was filled with farm animals.

Dandora was tranquil and beautiful despite its poverty. While visiting, I remembered some of the famous writing of the American author Henry David Thoreau, who chose to live in poverty to experience freedom from the busy world.

I became horrified at the harsh realities I was seeing in Africa, and I was losing my ability to think logically. I began to wish I could live in grassy Dandora indefinitely. I felt anger toward people I had grown up with for having extra money to spend on themselves when others had urgent needs. I told myself the people in Nairobi preferred living their simple lives in poverty. I soon wanted to become poor, quit school, and adopt lots of African children instead of completing my university education.

Through all of it, I felt content and deeply happy living in Africa. I think it was partly because of all of the new, special friends I made there so quickly and grew to love.

Perhaps I should have expected some Kenyan men I would meet during the summer would be interested in marrying an American like me. One afternoon, one of my male Kenyan friends who frequented the girls' home suggested that the two of us should get married. I reminded him that he had said he would never marry outside his tribe. He told me I was an exception. When I refused, he did not seem offended.

A few days after his proposal, the young man, some of the girls and I were walking Lakisama when an intoxicated man suddenly emerged from a small hut along the road. He approached me and grabbed my arm. Though the other girls tried to pull him off of me, we could not overpower him. After about a minute, a crowd of Kenyan children had gathered around us and began shouting for him to separate me from the other girls and assault me on the road in front of them. The crowd of children was closing in on us, and I was terrified. Rather than defending me, the Kenyan man who had proposed marriage made no effort to help.

At my moment of greatest danger, Naomi happened to be walking the area and saw what was happening. She was only a small woman, but she became enraged at the children and the intoxicated man. She was also shocked and angry at the young man for not helping me. When she loudly yelled at all of them, the children went away ashamed, and the man left me alone.

That summer another man followed me. He was living in Nairobi but was originally from the Congo. He spoke French and Swahili, but no English. He left me notes which had been translated into English by one of his friends, including a marriage proposal. Though I may have been in danger of him, neither he nor anyone else ever attacked me while I was living in Africa.

From the beginning of summer, I should have recognized that

living in Lakisama was unsafe for me. While in Lakisama, I wished I were a black Kenyan myself so I could blend in and be safe. I met many new friends all the time and loved walking all over the slums with them. I wanted to stay in the slums despite the danger.

I later found that my first African contact, the physician, who had suggested I live with Naomi, had never tried placing a Caucasian foreigner in that part of Lakisama before.

I should have asked Naomi to help me move to a safer location.

CHAPTER EIGHT

After a few days in Kenya, Naomi and some Kenyan friends traveled with me to downtown Nairobi so I could email my family. I also wanted to send an email to my Cleveland church that was financially supporting me. I determined I would tell my parents almost nothing about what I was seeing. I knew it would make them afraid.

I was beginning to think about my next trip, which I still hoped would be to West Africa, since it was another place where Susan had lived and spoken about. I thought about going to Southeast Asia after leaving Africa. I remembered my trip to China and my childhood desire to study Chinese. I later mentioned this to a church friend in an email, and he wrote back advising me to forget other trips and focus on living in Kenya.

After successfully writing friends and family and telling them I had arrived in Africa safely, I returned with Naomi to the slum.

§

While planning my trip to Africa, I had hoped to learn about the HIV epidemic there. I did not encounter HIV every day in Nairobi, but three of my friends' friends died suddenly. Their families said it was the flu or malaria, but experts I met told me with certainty that their deaths had been from HIV. Having HIV in Nairobi was considered embarrassing.

During my first couple weeks at the Lakisama medical clinic, I saw many horrible things. This included seeing a small child of about five with severe burns all over his body from his family's stove blowing up. He was in tremendous pain while a Kenyan nurse changed his bandages. I encountered other Kenyans who had been scarred, some for decades, with burns from stoves blowing up. But it was impossible for the poor to cook without the cheap stoves. They had no choice but to use them.

I still had big dreams of becoming a medical doctor. But on the day I encountered the child with the painful burns at the clinic, I reconsidered studying medicine. I did not want to see any more people in extreme pain. Instead, I wanted to find ways to get safer stoves to

Nairobi's poor for free or at a reduced cost. I wondered if raising money to purchase safer stoves and to meet other needs for Kenyan people could become a career opportunity for me.

I often thought about Susan's challenge to me not to go to Africa. She understood the heartache of encountering the poor who were suffering. Though I may have been delusional when I met her and saw her for much more than what she was, I found she was right. Nothing could have prepared me for what I encountered in Africa. My time there was emotionally devastating.

A couple of weeks into the summer, I went to downtown Nairobi with Naomi again. Since I checked email rarely in Africa, I received many messages from my parents who wanted badly to hear from me more often. They were extremely worried about my safety. I wrote my family a brief summary of what I was doing at the clinic and what I had seen, but I spent little time talking about my daily life. I told them how happy I was to have so many new friends. They thought I would be in a safe place, and I was not. I felt guilty.

Naomi eventually introduced me to some wealthy Kenyans. I found that my choice to live in the poor area often seemed ridiculous to wealthy Kenyan people, as well as Americans. I imagined the scenario in reverse, a wealthy Kenyan person visiting America and choosing to live in an area filled with American homeless people, like Skid Row in Los Angeles.

One Sunday, Naomi took me to Nairobi Chapel, a wealthy church in the nice area of downtown Nairobi. At the church, I met a wealthy Kenyan woman who was assisting the poor. Her name was Joyce.

Joyce explained how she and her husband had recently spent a substantial amount of money creating a Kenyan charity organization. Through her charity, she brought food and medicines to Timunu, a slum I had never seen. Joyce was a smart college graduate, and she had been a successful Nairobi businesswoman who made good money before establishing her charity.

I wanted to visit Joyce's charity in Timunu. After the church service, I decided to stay with Joyce's family for the night in their home and then drive to Timunu with Joyce the next day. I wanted to help Joyce any way I could. And I realized that staying in her family's home and visiting the slum by car would be safe.

Driving to Joyce's home in a car was a great relief after packing into the public transportation vans that Naomi, my impoverished friends and I had been using. I had already been in three old public vans in poor working condition that broke down in the slums.

§

Joyce's family lived in a quiet neighborhood that was filled with big plots of land and beautiful homes. Each of the homes had an enormous gate surrounding it. Their house had servants' quarters in front and extensive gardens in back. They had two other cars. Inside their home was a wooden spiral staircase, and the children's spacious rooms were upstairs. They had a color television, a landline phone, and two cell phones. Joyce gave me a private bedroom suite with a bath.

My parents badly wanted to know how they could reach me, and I regret that I did not give them Joyce's cell phone number. I felt my family would not approve of my situation entering dangerous slums every day, though I would generally be safe volunteering for Joyce's family, and living with them.

I was guilty and confused from the shock of living in wealth again with Joyce's family after living in Lakisama. Joyce understood the gap between Kenyan poverty and wealth, but I needed more help making sense of what I had seen than she was able to give.

§

Like other people I had met, Joyce thought that I had not been getting sufficient nutrition in the slum, and that I looked pale, even for a white person. During my first couple of weeks in Lakisama, I lived on grains, beans, other vegetables and tea, all in small quantities. But I did not think my friends in Lakisama seemed hungry or malnourished, and many were tall, strong and healthy. I did not know why I could not adjust to their food.

While living with Joyce's family, I began eating meat and

drinking milk again. Joyce and her husband noticed I regained the color in my face.

CHAPTER NINE

Reaching Timunu from Joyce's home took twenty minutes by car. When I arrived in Timunu, I saw about twenty Kenyan women in bright clothing socializing while they waited for Joyce. There was a big pot of porridge cooking on a fire outside a large concrete building.

Because Joyce's family personally sacrificed so much money to begin their new Nairobi charity, many of their Kenyan friends hated the guilt Joyce inadvertently made them feel. Some of her friends saw she was a CEO, and they encouraged Joyce to wear fancy leather boots and expensive, fashionable clothing to her small office in Timunu. She ignored their suggestions and wore casual dress, like me.

Many of the residents of Timunu were short on food. At the same time, they were smart, hardworking people. I had not yet met Kenyans who were short on food. What haunted me was that these people were forgotten, and their food shortage went unnoticed.

The charity Joyce had founded for the impoverished women and families of Timunu did not have a good website, and she asked if I might help with it, since she wanted support from America. She drove me to a Nairobi computer laboratory with an American-style coffee shop where I revised her website. As I worked on editing Joyce's online biography and objectives, I felt I was making a difference.

Joyce seemed to love having a white American like me interested in her work. We drove all over Nairobi together asking for donations for the women including medicines and hygienic products. As we drove to and from Timunu, Joyce explained how she was fundraising for the poor, including the details of her meetings with Nairobi corporations.

I came to love Joyce's children and husband, eating a big dinner every night with her family, and playing with her seven-year-old daughter, who loved to brush my auburn hair. When I decided to continue living in Joyce's home and volunteering in Timunu, Joyce charged me rent at a low rate. Her family was always generous.

I badly wanted to become like Joyce, a well-educated advocate for the poor with skill in leadership. I could see myself becoming someone like her.

§

I stayed with Joyce's family and volunteered in Timunu for a few more weeks, though I missed Naomi and the girls in Lakisama. While living with Joyce's family, I learned more about Kenyan and African politics from television and from newspapers. I had opportunities to hear economic, political and social discussions with Joyce's family and their well-educated friends.

I was introduced to a Rwandan man with a bachelor's degree in counseling, and his tall, beautiful Rwandan wife. I wanted to raise money in America to pay the Rwandan man to offer counseling services to his people in his home country. I thought of establishing an American charity. I wanted to employ African experts to work in their own countries.

§

After a few weeks living with Joyce's family, I decided I would return to Lakisama for a few days. Joyce and her husband were surprised that I wanted to go back. They knew it was extremely dangerous.

Despite the danger, I returned to Lakisama for a week near the end of the summer. I loved seeing the girls again. I spent a lot of time with Naomi, discussing her life and dreams. I rarely went places. I helped Naomi cook dinners and practice English with the girls. The girls taught me phrases in Swahili. One girl who lived in Naomi's home had Typhoid fever. I gave her a teddy bear.

After a week, I joined Naomi and two other Kenyan friends to travel to the city of Mombasa on Kenya's East Coast, and we all stayed with Naomi's friend for three days. We visited the white sands of the deep green Indian Ocean and museums on the coast.

Naomi and I traveled to a jungle an hour's drive from the city where she had other friends. When we arrived in the jungle, Naomi and I saw a small marketplace. I thought to myself that there would surely be no other Caucasians present, but only seconds later, I noticed a middle-aged white woman, perhaps a hundred feet in the distance. Years later, I wondered if my sighting of the white woman in the jungle was a hallucination. I still do not know. The sighting was possible, but unlikely, like many of the hallucinations I would experience years later.

I was happy to return to Nairobi, a city I had grown to love. But, immersed in the Kenyan culture, I had begun to love adventure. I traveled all over parts of Kenya that were considered unsafe for Americans to visit. It was hard not to want to see more of the country. The cities were vibrant and alive, filled with beautiful people who were proud to be dark skinned and to be Kenyan. I felt honored to live in their country.

§

During my last full week with Joyce's family, a Nigerian businessman named David visited Nairobi on business and spent a night in their home. Joyce and her husband had met David and his wife, Ruth, in America. They had all attended the National Prayer Breakfast years before.

I was excited to meet David. I told him I was an American college student studying molecular biology. I expressed how honored I would be to get to visit his country. I gave him a copy of some of my biochemistry research that was published. I saw David was a brilliant businessman with integrity. I wanted to meet Ruth.

That evening, David offered to host me in his family's home in Lagos, Nigeria for a week, but the Nigerian visa could only be obtained inside one's own country.

Later that night, David made a phone call to a political official he knew in Kenya. Because of his connection, I was granted an exception and was able to obtain my visa to Nigeria.

I had a feeling in my heart that my trip to Nigeria would be one of the most important of my life.

CHAPTER TEN

Since I had lived in Kenya for two months, I felt prepared to travel to Nigeria alone. On the plane to Lagos, I enjoyed seeing many black Africans in sophisticated, bright traditional West African dress. There were only a few other Caucasians on the plane, including a white family with a baby.

I met David at the airport. As we drove to his home, I saw a city that was huge, crowded and developed. I had no idea there were such wide and busy highway roads in Lagos. David and I traveled to his family's home on the highways in a fancy car with a hired driver. David was dignified and serious.

Each house within David's neighborhood was surrounded by its own double barbed wire. A servant was paged to open its huge gate, revealing an impressive, decorative, and large home. There were wood floors, pricey western- style furnishings, and impressive artwork.

I met Ruth, who was intelligent and lovely, and their delightful five-year-old daughter. I was given a large room with a private bath in the upstairs of their house. The view revealed some of the yard.

After a few minutes, Ruth called me on the phone in my bedroom to invite me to dinner. David's family had traveled far to bring me authentic American food, including ice cream and coffee. I loved their Nigerian food.

The next day David drove me to suburban areas with restaurants and large houses. He also drove me to a university where he introduced me to some university scientists, including a tall, smart female professor. Unfortunately, to reach our destinations, we often had to drive directly through areas of extreme poverty and neighborhoods filled with mud huts. Like Nairobi, the gap between the poor and the rich was wide. In Lagos, it seemed wider still.

David's family was providing HIV medications and testing kits at reasonable prices all over the West African region and was always doing honest business. He and Ruth cared greatly about their country's politics and economy, and about their country's poor.

§

I attended a Sunday church service in Lagos with David's family, and the dresses of the women were colorful and stunning. I found most cost $600-$800 American dollars. Many of the attendees loved to dance, and I felt welcomed into their warm and beautiful culture.

I went to an annual Christian conference in Lagos filled with both wealthy and impoverished Nigerians. I loved meeting more people and learning more about their lives, educations and customs. Since I was a white woman, and one of the only Caucasians present, conference leaders treated me like a celebrity. They gave me a spacious room and excellent food. Culture dictated that I not refuse the hospitality of my exemplary Nigerian hosts.

Encountering the poverty in Nigeria gave me a sense of gratitude for being an American that has stayed with me for all these years. And I still stand amazed at just how much a single family can do for their country. In Nigeria, I became better able to understand Susan, who had spent a month there.

I did not know that after spending one week in Nigeria, I would never be the same.

§

On my return to Nairobi, I stayed with Joyce's family for a few days before leaving Africa. I rested in Joyce's huge screen porch next to the gardens thinking about everything I had seen. I had developed a burning desire to get money to Africa, both the East and the West. I determined I wanted to raise funding for the Kenyan charities where I had volunteered and not go to medical school.

That summer I became aware that people with money and higher education could take a great stand for the poor in their societies, but I wanted to give away everything, including my money and my favorite possessions and clothes. It was not a logical solution or compassion. My mind was cloudy. My behavior was still changing.

When I boarded my flight from Addis Ababa to America, I told myself again that a life in poverty could be a wonderful life, like the wonderful lives of many happy, middle-class Americans.

Exhausted from the summer, I slept on the plane for many hours. While I was awake, I thought about the people I had grown to love in China, Kenya, and Nigeria.

§

I transferred planes in Washington D.C. after I returned to America. While in the capital, I met an uncle and his family, and stayed with them for a few days before I flew back to the university. I had no western style clothing, as I had left all of mine in Nigeria as a gift.

While with my uncle's family, I could talk about nothing but Africa, and I had an enormous amount of energy. My odd behavior must have been obvious to my uncle and aunt.

On my return to America, I did not debrief with anyone with international experience or ask anyone to give me advice about reentering America. This was a big mistake. Susan had debriefed with a knowledgeable American family who had traveled extensively when she returned from Africa. It was how I met her.

But I probably would not have listened to advice anyway. I thought I needed no help making sense of what I had seen. And the pain I felt from what I had encountered was so intense and deep that it would have been excruciating to share it with a counselor.

If I had been mentally healthy upon my return from Africa, I would have recommitted myself to coursework with renewed motivation. I should have studied hard to become better qualified to raise money for Africa. But when I returned from Africa, I was not the same person I had been before I traveled there.

§

I flew back to the university after visiting my uncle and aunt in Washington D.C. I was to begin my senior year of college. My new university apartment was on the sixth floor and had a lovely view. I liked my new roommate, who was also scheduled to graduate in the spring.

But on my return, as I unpacked a lot of jewelry that was given to me during my childhood and teenage years, I felt guilty to hold onto it. I began giving it away to friends who did not care about it. As a teenager, I loved gold jewelry, and I had some small, valuable pieces that were many years old, and held special memories for me. They used to be my treasures.

The first African friend I met at the airport in Ethiopia had worn a gold chain and felt no shame. She explained to me that the gold was appropriate in situations where she was raising money for causes she believed in, like raising money for her adopted children. I had encountered Naomi, Joyce and David, who taught me how much good a person with money can do, and how rich people can become advocates for the poor. But I forgot everything.

One day, back in America, I took one of my gold necklaces I had received from my family for a birthday and threw it away. I still do not know exactly why I did it, but it had something to do with seeing Africa and something to do with my mind failing me. More and more often, my thinking was not making sense. I wanted to distance myself from family and friends who valued their possessions more than the international problem of poverty. In addition to throwing away one of my gold necklaces, I threw away other jewelry, clothes and some of my favorite books.

Something inside of me was wrong. Soon after I returned from Africa, I fell apart.

CHAPTER ELEVEN

I was scheduled to graduate with my bachelor's degree in molecular biology in the spring of 2003. I was excited to be almost finished. But upon my return from Africa, I was constantly reflecting on what I had seen, and I could not rest.

From 1999 to 2002, my parents made financial sacrifices to pay for me to attend college. They wanted me to be immersed in my love and passion for learning, and to realize my dreams of doing research or going to medical school. I used to love the beautiful university I attended, and the excitement I felt there.

My parents were eager to get tickets to my graduation, and they invited me to return with them to Ohio after my graduation, to stay with them while I looked for a job. They did not know how deeply traumatized and confused I had become while living in Africa.

I knew the best way to prepare to fundraise for Africa was to attend medical school or enter a Ph.D. program. I knew I needed to focus and get my best grades during my senior year to prepare for my future. But against everyone's advice, I decided to set up a small American nonprofit organization as soon as I returned to the university.

I found a small group of friends, mostly students, who were interested in my ideas to create a nonprofit organization. I contacted Naomi in Africa and other international people to ask if they would be on our board of directors. I planned to fly people from all over the world to attend a board meeting. I never thought of how I might pay for their airfare.

I had the idea of beginning an online biological research journal. I was not qualified to establish a research journal, but I knew people from my former research who were qualified. I discussed with others how I might collect research from remote parts of the world. Though I had not finished my undergraduate degree, I began to talk like I already had a Ph.D., and like I was qualified to establish the journal.

I planned to complete paperwork to incorporate my new charity and to apply for tax-exempt status while I studied for classes that fall, 2002. During the first semester of my freshman year, I studied hard and made good grades while working many hours in research. This time, I hoped to work on the nonprofit organization while I was studying.

§

Before fall classes began, I had spent many hours online reading about how to incorporate a charity. I had a few friends who believed in me and helped me with the incorporation papers and the application for tax-exemption. I enjoyed completing the paperwork for a cause I believed in. But as the first weeks of the fall semester passed by, spending time filling out paperwork became my priority over my courses. I had never wanted the charity to take priority over my coursework. But I could not focus on my classes. I had the problem before, but never to this extent. I spent time emailing friends from Africa and other countries.

That fall, I took an advanced genetics class. After I turned in the first exam, I was certain I had a perfect score. I remembered how I had received perfect scores on exams before while in college. But I failed the exam.

I could not believe what was happening. It was like a nightmare. I soon found that whenever I tried to study, I could not focus on anything but my memories of Africa and my plans to fundraise. I found myself unable to pass exams in any of my classes.

Deep inside, I knew something was very wrong. I was no longer capable of studying.

§

I was in denial about the suffering I had seen in Africa, and would be for years after my return. Sometimes, in fall of 2002, I began telling American friends that Africa was the loveliest and most wonderful place I had ever seen. I still thought about how the people in the slums of Nairobi and mountains of China sometimes seemed happy and content like many people in America.

I never had nightmares or flashbacks about the miseries I had witnessed in Africa. But on my return, I could not stop thinking of the suffering I had seen. I was unable to cope with the reality of the poverty I encountered.

A few weeks into the semester my mind had not improved, and I still could not study. I hoped that, somehow, if I did not drop my classes, the professors would never actually give me F's. I did not drop any of my classes.

After returning from Africa, I became even more obsessed with traveling. I began to think about sending funds to poor people in other countries besides the African countries I visited, like Thailand. There were Americans living in Thailand who I used to know through my old church. I decided to write and ask if I might visit them in Thailand over my Christmas break. I wanted to meet Thai charity representatives and collect information about them. I hoped that I might send money to Thailand as well as Africa.

I became obsessed with the idea of traveling to Thailand. I planned to invite a group of people to come to Thailand with me. There were seven people I hoped would join me. But I had no plans for how I might raise enough money to bring along other people. I considered selling an old violin, but I could not part with it at that time.

I had no success in inviting others to come with me. I decided to travel alone.

As I planned to go to Southeast Asia again, my mind was fuzzy in a way it had never been in my life. I had no time to rest after returning to America from Africa. In October, things had not changed. As I was failing college, I convinced myself I did not have time for both my classes and the new nonprofit. I told myself the nonprofit was the reason I was failing, and that the nonprofit was my higher priority. I was in this state of mind when I planned to go to Thailand.

§

From my childhood until I began studying at the university, I had almost never had anyone tell me I was wrong about any major decision. I had always been a "perfect" child and never caused any problems. I excelled in school. My freshman year of college, my parents felt I should work fewer hours in the research laboratory, so I might concentrate on my classes, and so I could socialize more with other students. Though I was not willing to listen to their advice about school and friendships, the issues we disagreed about were minor. Whenever I *was* wrong, I could not see it.

When my friends and family told me they did not agree with my decision to travel again, at first, I thought they were persecuting me. I thought of Mother Teresa. I considered my upcoming trip to Thailand to be a wise choice coming from the best of myself. I knew that Mother Teresa had no college degree. Though my parents greatly disapproved of my decision to travel to Thailand, I was single-minded about traveling again. I believed my travels were part of a divine mission to do good in my world.

§

That fall, I needed to get my driver's license renewed. Rather than visiting my parents, I flew to visit old friends from my hometown near Cleveland, and I used their address on my license. My friends were concerned about the disagreement I had with my parents over my upcoming Thailand trip. While I was in Cleveland, a group of my family's friends, most in their forties, arranged a meeting and met with me while my parents were on speakerphone. Most of them were my parents' age. They wanted to help me reconcile with my parents, and encouraged me to cancel my next trip to Southeast Asia. But I would not alter my plans to travel. I clung to my plans. I saw old friends and my family as heartless.

On my return to the university from Cleveland, when I was still planning to visit Thailand, my mom called to say that she and my dad would withdraw their financial support unless I canceled my trip.

I did not share with them that I was doing poorly in school. I knew it would have made them heartbroken. No one understood that I had in fact been trying my best in school. I still did not even realize myself that I truly could not study. I did not tell many people that I thought I was part of a divine mission. My parents and I did not understand each other. I felt misunderstood by everyone.

I visited my bank and found that I was eligible for a loan big enough to allow me to pay for both my tuition and living expenses. I could graduate on time without my parents' support. I was confident that I could both visit Thailand and finish my studies. I decided to relinquish my parent's financial support.

But perhaps I did not realize my trip was not their greatest concern. The biggest problem was that I had an arrogant attitude, and I thought I was perfect. I never really tried to communicate my thoughts to my parents with humility and explain that I believed I was capable of both studying hard and traveling. Traveling looked great on my university resume and was encouraged by the university. I never invited my parents to see my trip to Thailand the way that I saw it.

When my parents stopped financially supporting me, I took out a large loan to pay for finishing my senior year classes so I could graduate. I arranged to move into a cheaper university apartment. After I decided to travel rather than receive my parents' financial support, I refused to speak to them.

§

A few weeks after I signed paperwork for the large loan, I still could not pull myself together and concentrate. I realized the loan money I had taken was giving me time to work on the nonprofit while I lived in the university apartment.

That October as I bought plane tickets to travel to Southeast Asia, my parents' disapproval sometimes made me wonder if my parents and their friends truly believed in God. I began to see my kind and loving parents as people without compassion.

I realized that if my parents were in my life, they might actually work against my goals of raising money for the poor, trying to force me to return to school instead. I felt I needed to protect my future plans by breaking off all contact with them. I decided to stop reading their emails and answering their phone calls. I completely cut them off.

I remembered passages in the Bible where Jesus said those who followed him were his true family. I noticed that a couple running a charity in Thailand had the same first names as some of my relatives. I wondered if the couple who were running the charity were my "true family." It seemed to me that God was providing new friends in place of my parents, other relatives and old friends.

During the next few weeks, which included my twenty-first birthday, I still refused all contact from my parents. On my birthday, they tried to call and ask what address they should send my twenty-first birthday present to, but I did not return their call. I had become completely incapable of relating normally with friends and family.

During my time as a college student, I heard about a university philosophy professor who was known as a humanitarian. I had met with him once before my trip to Africa. In October, I went to his office and showed him my passport stamps from East and West Africa. I asked him for advice on raising money. He seemed to believe in me, and he encouraged me in my efforts to fundraise for the poor. He had no idea I had problems balancing college life with my new ambition, and was becoming alienated from family and friends.

I met with another professor at the university several times. He discussed international politics with me, including what I had seen in Africa and China. He also encouraged me, and he seemed interested in my plan for creating a new nonprofit organization. Both professors had no reason to believe I was not a normal or even a high-achieving student. I had been in the past. Working hard on my charitable endeavor, I was utilizing university resources and meeting university professors while failing my classes. I believed what I was doing was good and right.

The deterioration happening in my mind was affecting my life in other ways. I became uninterested in my most precious possessions. I finally decided to sell my dearest possession, my violin, to raise funds for Africa. The decision was irrational. That fall, I found a local violin dealer and eventually sold the violin for a small fraction of its worth. I donated all of the money from its sale to my charity.

Before going to Africa, I had placed almost all of my belongings, except for my jewelry, in a small house owned by an elderly woman from my church. Her home was a walking distance from the university. After I returned from Africa, she tried to contact me, but I was irresponsible, and I went several months without being in touch with her. Finally, she went through everything I owned, giving or throwing my things away. I lost almost everything as though I had suffered through a fire.

During the entire fall of 2002, my state of mind was as though I had heard news that a loved one had suddenly and unexpectedly died, and I never recovered from the shock. My mind was in a growing state of confusion and sadness all the time. It was becoming more and more cloudy.

§

After returning from Africa in 2002, and before going to Thailand, I met an American girl a little younger than I was, Danielle, who wanted to visit Africa. I helped Danielle prepare to travel to Nairobi to live near where I had stayed but in a safer location. It was exciting to help Danielle plan her trip to Kenya. She later returned with many pictures. On her return, she was changed and inspired by her visit to Africa.

Danielle invited me to her home in the southwest United States so we could discuss what we had seen in Nairobi. The trip was an expression of thanks because I helped to plan her trip. Danielle generously paid for my airfare to visit her. The two of us talked about what we had seen in Africa. She was making long-term plans to return to Africa after her graduation.

On Danielle's return from Africa, she did not struggle with losing her concentration, and she did not act strangely like me. She recognized what a difference she might make in Africa with a college degree. Danielle studied hard and finished her bachelor's degree.

But even when she graduated and I had not, I still felt I was special. When I saw she had finished her degree, I was too detached from reality to regret not finishing my own.

§

By November 2002, I had lost all touch with my family, from phone calls to emails, and they had little idea where I was or what I was doing. My parents tried sending me checks to make sure I had some financial support. I was worried they would use the gifts to get back into my life, so I did not cash them. Perhaps I was paranoid. But I knew that if they were in my life, they would mandate I get a job or return to school, and in my heart, I knew I was no longer capable of either.

I did not want my parents to know the address of the new apartment I was going to move into in late November, so I established a private mailbox near the university campus. I stopped using my residence address and used the personal mailbox as my permanent address.

Weeks went by, and my mind became even more foggy. I still could not stand to hear from my parents. Whenever they sent me mail, I would immediately rip it up. My mom liked putting little animals and smiley faces on the envelopes. But all I could see was that they did not want to give away all their money to people who I loved in Africa.

After I was not responding to their letters, my parents sent a beautifully wrapped package to my church. It was a large package and decorated with bunny stickers. But when I heard from my church that my parents sent me something, I was angry, and I asked that the package be returned. My friends at the church did not understand why I wanted it returned. Years before, perhaps my heart would have melted. I was losing not only my mind, but my heart.

§

That fall, I never explained to anyone that I was failing my classes. Everyone in my life encouraged me to continue school and obtain a Ph.D. I had planned to earn a Ph.D. In the past, I had been as certain about getting a Ph.D. or medical degree as most teenagers are about graduating from high school.

I was reluctant to speak with friends about my future. At times, I went along with their conversations about doing a Ph.D. even though I was failing my undergraduate courses. This was deceptive, but I did not know what to say. I still believed I was doing what was right. I believed I could study if I wanted to. I was certain that my choices were appropriate, but I recognized that others would see them as wrong, so I felt my lies were justified.

Knowing there were others who believed in my nonprofit encouraged me. Though I had almost no money, I still planned to fly my international friends to the university area for a board meeting. I hoped it would happen later in 2003. Some who I asked to be board members I barely knew.

I had always enjoyed meeting international students on campus. On my return from Africa, I asked some of them to meet me and speak with me on a few occasions to discuss the cultures of their countries and their countries' poor. I talked with them about my own travels. After meeting each of these people, I listed them as members of my organization on the new website. I cannot remember if I asked them for permission before listing them. I do remember that most were happy to talk with me and to be involved in my work in a small way. I believed I would someday send money to poor people in the home countries of all of these students.

§

That fall, I decided I would never speak to my parents again for the rest of my life. I believed they had no hearts and were not true Christians. I noticed that many families had divisions. I considered my division from them to be necessary and normal.

I purchased my ticket to Thailand in late October 2002. I would stay in Thailand for three weeks and then in Hong Kong for one week on vacation. To purchase the tickets, I nearly maxed out two credit cards. I was certain that someone who believed in me would later come along and pay off all of my debt, including my university debt. As for my credit debt, someone later did.

My parents continued to write long letters that I did not read and made phone calls that I did not answer. I was flooded with email from church friends from home in Ohio. Some had known me for over a decade and cared deeply about me. When they heard from my parents that something was wrong, they wanted to help.

After receiving emails from these people, I used the block feature on my email account to never hear from them again. I was afraid that if I read the messages, I would be drawn in and not emotionally strong enough to remain estranged from my parents. I hoped to never hear from any of them again, and I never read any of their email. One day, I became tired of the repeated phone messages I received every day from my worried parents. I unplugged my phone.

Weeks prior, I had asked my parents if we might meet on Thanksgiving of 2002 rather than Christmas because I hoped to be in Southeast Asia during Christmas. When I refused to speak with my parents, my brother tried writing me. He informed me that my parents had purchased tickets for me to visit them during Thanksgiving. I never wrote my parents or brother accepting or rejecting the flight. I worried that contact with my brother might bring me to speak with my parents, and I lost touch with him. Meanwhile, every day, I daydreamed about the best ways I might raise money and send it overseas. I hoped to make wealthy connections in America.

In November, I convinced myself I could do without my college degree. I told myself that the coursework was below my level of intelligence and a waste of time. When I realized I would be receiving F's, I told myself that I was like Bill Gates and other famous people who did not complete college degrees. I knew I could still become super successful without graduating from college. I believed the F's would somehow work to give me a brighter future.

Even though I had dropped out, I signed up for spring classes during November. I paid for my spring classes using the large loan I took out in October. I registered for four classes, including two I had already taken at the community college years prior. The two classes were supposed to transfer but did not. I thought I would be learning nothing. In high school, I loved learning new things and taking many diverse classes, but I never remembered that time of my life. Instead, I planned my trip to Southeast Asia.

§

I had been fascinated with life and culture in the Middle East for years. I had known several people through the university from the Middle East, and others who had visited or lived in many Middle Eastern countries. As I traveled to China and Africa, I became fascinated with the cultures in other places I had never visited. A month before leaving for Thailand, I began planning a trip to visit the Middle East.

In retrospect, it was inappropriate for me to plan a trip to the Middle East at that time. In one year, I had gone to China and Africa and was planning to go to Thailand. But I planned the trip anyway.

That November, I found another student who was interested in visiting the Middle East. We planned to travel together during the university's spring break, 2003. The two of us applied to a university program that offered grants for student projects, seeking funds to travel to the Middle East. I printed out my itinerary from America to Egypt. After applying for funding, my friend and I won payment of half of our airfare to and from Egypt.

During the fall, I did everything in my power to obtain visas for Middle Eastern countries I wanted to visit, including Saudi Arabia. But certain laws had changed. Though I was able to get a visa to Egypt, I could not obtain visas to a few other countries.

A few weeks after winning the funding, a university professor called me to say that it was extremely dangerous to travel to the Middle East at that time. He said that the money we had been granted was a mistake. He encouraged my friend and me to visit a different part of the world.

Through all of this, the university was apparently not aware I had dropped out of my classes. Perhaps this was because my failing grades had not been finalized yet. I was using my student status to work on university computers, spend countless hours on nonprofit paperwork, and obtain funding for my trip to the Middle East. I continued meeting and talking with professors who thought I was a student.

I hoped to travel to Egypt and then to visit an embassy there to try to get visas to other Middle Eastern countries. Because of the danger, my friend no longer wanted to travel with me. I hoped to travel to the Middle East alone during the university's spring break. I did not bother to ask for money from the student committee again. I did not know how I would pay for the trip, but I believed somehow it would just work out.

CHAPTER TWELVE

My host family in Thailand had lived in the country for about two years. Prior to that, they lived near the university where they attended my church. My junior year, they had encouraged me to go to China. During the time I knew them, my mind had changed, and I became a different person.

Before I left for Thailand, my friends there contacted me and recommended I wait to travel until my graduation. I ignored their advice. I was insistent on coming to Thailand immediately. I believed my sense of urgency to visit them was divine, though I did not tell them that. I continued to hope that my trip to Thailand would make me more like Mother Teresa.

The day before I flew to Thailand, I emailed the family there who would host me and let them know I had dropped out of school. I felt my decision to drop out had been right. I flew to Thailand without checking if they had replied.

§

In December 2002 I went to visit Thailand, Myanmar and Hong Kong. My trip did not go as planned.

I purchased tickets to Thailand with a transfer in Hong Kong, and I planned to stay in China for a week after visiting Thailand. When I first arrived in Hong Kong, it was eleven at night, and my layover there was eighteen hours. I needed a hotel room for the night. There was a hotel conveniently located beside the airport, but it was too expensive for me. Instead, I went to a side area of the airport to lie down for the night on some airport chairs.

I was surprised at how many other people were spending the night in the airport, though I saw no other women or children. Everyone appeared to be a white businessman except for one man. He looked disheveled and dirty, but appeared to be comfortable and in a deep sleep. He looked to me like a homeless person within the airport.

That night, I fell into a light sleep, but woke up at least once every hour. I was close to a Hong Kong airline's service desk. At midnight, I saw an airline staff member use a dry mop to dust off a huge sign with the airline's name, which I cannot remember. From five to six A.M., airline workers began to flood into the airport and open shops serving coffee and selling souvenirs and newspapers. The sunrise revealed mountains in the distance. After a horrible night, the view was lovely.

When airport personnel arrived, I watched a Chinese woman wake up the disheveled man I noticed before. She was angry to see him asleep there and forced him to wake up and move away from her shop. It seemed she had seen him before. I wondered how and when he arrived and whether he was homeless. I wondered what might happen to him.

After the long night, I stayed in the Hong Kong airport until the mid-afternoon, when I boarded my flight to Bangkok. It was the longest day of my life.

Perhaps I was dressed inappropriately in the Bangkok airport, with my waist-long light brown hair freely flowing, and bright red lipstick. I did not know my appearance would make me a target for men. An Asian man approached me and deliberately stepped into my path to get my attention. The incident startled me. I tried to get an earlier flight to my destination in the west of Thailand. I was successful, and I arrived an hour early to meet my host family.

§

At the airport in western Thailand, my host family was happy to see me, but I did not know what a great burden I would be to them. Because I had not given them my exact arrival time, they did not know exactly when to expect me, or if I was even coming at all. As I flew to Southeast Asia, I continued telling myself that collecting information about the international poor was a greater priority than my college graduation.

From my first day in Thailand, my host family did not understand what had happened to the dream I used to have of becoming a research scientist. They saw I had changed. I was not interested in their lives, their friends, their church, or even seeing the city. We spent Christmas Day together. They gave me presents, but I do not remember giving them anything. They invited me to go to a Thai theatre and watch a *Lord of the Rings* movie with them on Christmas Day (though I was too restless to enjoy the movie). They welcomed me to walk around Bangkok with them over the holidays.

Though they were always kind to me, I did not appreciate it. I regret that I took them out to eat only once to thank them for hosting me. I never offered to pay them rent for my stay, which lasted about three weeks. While living with them, I began learning to ride their motorcycle and accidently lost their helmet. After I returned to America, I could not remember losing it, so I did not offer to pay for it or replace it. It was worth about $50.

My whole time in Thailand, I constantly bothered my host family, demanding we meet as many Thai charities as possible. They did everything they could to introduce me to missionaries and aid workers while I was in Thailand. This included the family who ran a medical clinic in a rural area and had the same names as my relatives. I loved the clinic, and I wanted to send the clinic funding when I returned to America, in addition to the funding I hoped to send to Africa. After meeting members of the Thai medical clinic, I believed my trip had been successful.

Before I left Thailand, my kind host family expressed their heartfelt concern that I had dropped out of my classes, but I was unresponsive. I felt they did not understand. I still believed I was a straight-A student if I wanted to be. I thought I was perfect. Since my host family had expressed disapproval that I dropped out of school, I felt I needed to cut them off, and on my return to America, I would block all the emails they would send me.

§

After three weeks in Thailand, I arrived in Hong Kong again. This time, I left the airport, taking a train to meet the sister of a friend from the university. The goal of my Hong Kong trip was to vacation in the city and see the prominent buildings and attractions, and had nothing to do with visiting the poor or fundraising. My host in Hong Kong was generous, and she gave me a key to her small apartment. I was free to go wherever I wanted while she worked. On the evenings and weekends, we toured the city together. At the end of my trip, I had fallen in love with Hong Kong, and I did not want to leave China. I wanted to live there for years.

Back in America, I had almost no money left. I used the rest of what was available on my credit cards to withdraw cash, deposit it, and mail a check to the Thai charity.

When I returned to America, I was even more zealous to find financial support for clinics I visited in Africa and in Thailand. I had no plan to attend classes, but I used the loan I had taken to pay for four spring semester classes while I continued living in my university apartment. I was delusional, believing I still might graduate. I never attended the four classes.

In January 2003 it had been three months since I spoke with my parents. I thought every day of the suffering I had seen in Nairobi, my experiences in China, and of the small clinic in northern Thailand. My memories of the international poor never faded as I continued to dodge letters and phone calls from my parents, other family members, and friends. I rarely thought about my family.

One day, a university housing resident assistant came by to check on me. She seemed tremendously worried about me, and she spoke to me slowly and looked at me as though I were crazy. She asked a few questions about my classes, but I was unresponsive, so she left.

I knew that under the umbrella of university housing, parents were welcome to call the resident assistants and make sure their sons and daughters were doing well. After my encounter with the resident assistant, I realized that my parents were definitely going to come to the university soon and find me out. I imagined my parents wanted to know what was happening in my life. I was afraid of seeing them because I knew I was not capable of returning to school. I was offended that the resident assistant was meddling in my life.

That January, I had become as mentally incapable of working as I was of taking classes. I still believed that not going to school or doing any other work was my choice, and not because I was unable. I knew that if I were in touch with my parents, they would mandate that I either attend classes or get a job. In my heart, I still knew I was incapable of doing either.

I continued to use the nonprofit as an excuse. I believed in my mission to do good in the world, and that I was making my life choices as a Christian. I wanted to emulate the lives of Gandhi and Jesus.

I believed my separation from my parents was necessary. I did not drink, do drugs, or engage in sexual activity. I had committed no crime. I always tried to be respectful. I believed I was making right choices.

And through all of it, to this day, I have never shared my expectations of becoming rich and famous with anyone. There is no need, because when it happens, everyone will see.

§

One day in early March of 2003, I had a dream that my parents were let into my apartment by the university staff, and that my parents were infuriated as they had never been before. The dream led me realize that if my parents knew I had dropped out of school, they would be angry and confused. I woke up to the reality that if I were to stay in university housing, my parents would come find me. I believed my parents would try to work with the university and pressure me into returning to school. In my heart, I knew that my best efforts produced failing grades.

I began to fear that if we were in touch, my parents would poison my name to students interested in hearing about my trip to Africa who were considering helping me raise money for the clinics. I believed that raising money for the poor overseas was my personal mission from God and the most important work in my life.

That morning, I told my roommates that if anyone they did not know were to come to see me, they were not to let them in.

CHAPTER THIRTEEN

I had committed to pay monthly rent for the rest of the school year, about a thousand dollars total. Though legally obligated, I did not have the money to pay. But on March 3, 2003, I made the decision to live nowhere rather than be found in my university apartment by friends and family. I took the few possessions I had to the apartment of a responsible friend. I stashed my things in a closet, and my friend offered to let me keep them there indefinitely.

After storing my possessions, I turned in the key to my university apartment to the housing office. Then, carrying only a small bag with a few changes of light clothing, and some small toiletries, I left the apartment complex forever.

I was unsure where I would be spending that night. I thought of my ticket itinerary to Egypt. I was to fly there with a plane transfer in Boston. I began to believe that if I were in Boston, thousands of miles from the university, I would be safe from my family. I believed that in Boston, someone would come to the airport, meet me, and give me money to send to Africa and Thailand. I was unsure of exactly how much money the person would give, or for the poor in what country. I wondered if the person might pay for my trip to Egypt, have connections in the Middle East, or tell me where I might stay there. I expected this person I was to meet at the airport was a man, and that I might even marry him.

§

March 3, 2003 was my first day without keys to a home, and without anywhere to stay. I went to the travel agency and had my itinerary changed to the same day. I had already paid for a round trip ticket to Boston, but not to Egypt. The $50 charge to change my ticket cost me nearly all of my remaining money.

A university friend from my old church, Scott, was willing to take me to the airport. He did not know exactly why I was leaving my classes to travel so suddenly. He had certainly heard rumors of my issues with my family. But he ignored whatever he had heard and kindly offered to drop me off at the airport. As we drove there, I discussed the significance of the day, March 3, 2003, three-three-three. I felt the day was lucky.

While boarding the plane to Boston, I felt great relief to be out of the university area, and out of my apartment. By going to Boston, I was away from the resident advisor who had begun to ask questions. I had sensed that I would encounter my parents again soon, so I needed to get away. Boarding the plane to Boston, I remembered the faces of the African people whom I loved and for whom my heart was broken. I believed this was a necessary step in my life to help them.

§

After arriving in Boston, I went to an airport help desk, and I asked the airport worker which organizations were available to assist students traveling to remote areas of the world to help the poor. The woman seemed to want to help, but she had never heard of such a network of people. Since I had not been in touch with my parents since October 2002, and had no paying job, I found myself in Boston with less than $50 in my bank account. I had already maxed out my credit cards. I had only a $20 bill in my pocket.

The morning I arrived in Boston, I found a small chapel in the airport. I sat in the chapel for a while, and then at noon a service began, which I enjoyed. There were many wealthy travelers and business people at the service, and I met a few of them. I gave a middle-aged businessman a business card I had created for myself with my new charity's name.

After the service, I went to meet the minister. I casually mentioned to him that I was traveling and had lost some money. I inquired about a place to stay for the night.

The minister was one of the rudest people I have ever encountered during my life. He first seemed friendly and led me to his office to talk, but when I inquired about a place to stay, he abruptly entered his office and forcefully slammed the office door in my face, making me feel like trash. At the beginning of my time without a place to stay, and after I spoke with him, I realized that my homelessness had to be a secret. I learned that if my secret were revealed, I would be treated in a way I would never have imagined could happen in America. I saw that if anyone found out I was homeless, my research publications, violin honors, good grades, and all other abilities became nothing. It was like I was no longer a person.

During the first few hours in the Boston airport, no one came to ask me if I needed help, offered to host me, or gave me money to send overseas. I was certain that any person could have had a dream about me and woken up knowing where I was. I reasoned that someone could even learn in a dream that they were supposed to come to meet me and marry me. I eagerly waited for the person who I believed would be a "savior" to me. But as the hours went by, no one came.

I spent the night on a chair in the Boston airport. I felt certain it was impossible for my parents and friends to locate me, and this gave me relief. My mental state kept me from seeing what I was doing. I was beginning to be somewhat catatonic. I was sitting, thinking and daydreaming in the airport for hours on end.

There was a huge difference between how I felt in the Hong Kong airport, awake nearly all night, and how I felt that night in Boston. In Boston, with my cloudy mind, I was able to sleep comfortably in an airport chair for the entire night. I never thought back to the man I saw in the Hong Kong airport who appeared homeless or realized that I was behaving like he was. Unlike my time in Hong Kong, the hours in Boston went by quickly.

§

The next morning, when I woke up at the airport, I realized I had been there for over fifteen hours. I was hungry, and I bought a couple of donuts with my $20 bill. I realized that no one was coming to the airport to take me home with them. My choices were to either enter a homeless shelter in Boston or to fly back to the university area and stay with friends. The option of going to stay with my parents or their friends never entered my mind.

I went to the airline kiosk to change my flight and return to the university out west. But changing my flight cost about $50, and the airline staff would not accept a combination of my cash plus money from my bank account. Since my credit cards had been maxed out, I was unable to pay for the ticket to be changed.

I did not know what to do. Finally, I thought of my friend from my old university church who was allowing me to store some of my things in his closet. I had known him for years. During my sophomore and junior years, I invited him and other friends to my apartment for dinners and parties. I decided to call him.

I used the change from my $20 bill to make the call on an airport payphone. He answered. In broken words, I began to explain my situation to him. But my friend required no explanation and asked no questions. He immediately called the airport and paid for my ticket change to fly me back. After changing my ticket, he called me back on the airport payphone to make sure I was okay.

§

While boarding the plane to return to the west, I was wearing an expensive jacket decorated with the name and insignia of the university of which I was a dropout. Another passenger asked me if I was a student there, and I excitedly told him I was. I was still proud of the university, and confused.

When I had flown back from Boston, my friend who paid the $50 for my return trip invited me to his house, which he shared with a few students. I had dressed up to meet the people I believed were going to come meet me in Boston, and I was wearing a nice long black wool skirt and fancy shirt with nylons, though my nylons had torn. I had not showered in a couple of days, though I still looked good. My friend and the students living with him offered me a shower. That night, he spent the night sleeping in his living room so I could sleep in his bedroom by myself.

I slept well at my friend's house. I was grateful to finally be back from my disappointment in Boston. A few days later, I pooled my cash money with the money in my checking account, and I wrote my friend a check to cover the ticket change expense. He never cashed it.

At the end of the Boston trip, I did not abandon my hope that someday a "savior" would come and support my charity work. Instead, I felt the need to wait for the "savior" to come, and I was sure he would someday. Even after my experience in Boston, I did not contact my family. I was running from my parents and old friends as though they were dangerous thieves who wanted to harm me and stop me from achieving my goals.

Although I was slowly slipping into a more foggy state of mind, I was not bothering anyone. I was still maintaining decent hygiene. I knew that if people discovered I was homeless I would be treated like trash as I was in Boston, so I decided to never tell anyone the details of my living situation. I wanted to look and act like everybody else.

§

After I returned from Boston, I needed to find how I could get food and where I could sleep. Though he had been kind, I could not continue staying with my friend. Perhaps I should have gone back to university housing office where I had turned in my key and say it had been a mistake. I was still obligated to pay rent for the next two months, until the end of the semester, though I was no longer living there.

After I returned from Boston, I felt desperate to conceal the truth about my living arrangements and status in school. I never considered telling anyone I had lost my mind, if that was even what was happening. I wondered if I would someday earn an honorary Ph.D. from my international fundraising work. I wondered if I were a prophet. I never shared these thoughts with anyone. I still reasoned that when I became successful, everyone would see.

I began telling new people I met that I was a part-time graduate student. I thought it was half true. During my undergraduate studies, I had done graduate-level research. My molecular biology research had been published twice, and my third paper was about to be printed.

§

I decided to contact the family of my old roommate from the summer after my freshman year. I had spent time with her family that summer when I was missing my own family, and the family lived only a half hour from campus. In early March, I asked them for a place to rest for a few days, giving few details. They invited me to stay at their house indefinitely.

While I was living with the family, I was able to rest and think about Africa and Thailand, and my goals of sending money. I thought about the friends I made in America who wanted to help (though most of them were international students who were only my acquaintances). Though I had almost no money of my own, I still felt confident that raising money for the poor was what I was supposed to do. I did not know that, soon, I would have success that would be worth waiting for.

§

After spending a few days as a guest of the family, I knew I could not stay any longer at their home. They were kind to me, and the time had been wonderful, but I did not want to intrude. Before I left, the family offered to help with my nonprofit, but since they were old enough to be my parents, I was afraid they would take over my organization. I refused their help. My fear made no sense and was based on nothing.

After my stay, my old roommate's mom drove me back to the university area. I felt revived and ready for the next phase of my life, though I did not know what it would be.

§

I called one more family from my old church and asked for their help. They lived only a short walk from the university. I did not know them well, but we had many mutual friends. I showed them the Power Point presentation some friends and I created for my new nonprofit. They encouraged me to continue my work.

I stayed with the family for a few days. One evening, I told them I was apprehensive about seeing my family, but I was ambiguous in my explanations of why. When I told them how I felt, they plainly advised me to get a warrant to prevent my parents from seeing me again. But they did not really understand my situation. If they had known what had really happened, they would not have suggested it. Even with my confused mind, I was certain that getting a court order to keep my parents away was wrong.

The second family I visited was interested in helping me get funding to finish my bachelor's degree. When I told them about my goals to raise money, they felt that finishing my schooling was a higher priority. They wanted to help. I believe that if I expressed a desire to return to the university, they would have personally made it possible for me. Of course, if I had decided to return to school, I could have contacted my own family, who probably would still have helped me graduate. It was not what I wanted.

I began to convince myself that the reason I was not graduating was because my parents stopped supporting me. This was ridiculous. I had already taken out a loan to be able to finish my classes and graduate. I thought of many reasons why I was not finishing school, always telling myself I could have if I had wanted to.

Before I left the second family's home, and in an effort to encourage me, they narrated a true story to me. They said that one of their acquaintances from a church believed his calling was to live with the homeless. Though the man did not consider himself to be a homeless person, he began living under a bridge with homeless people. He believed that the area under the bridge was his "post." The man's decision to become homeless stayed with me for many years. It was the first time I had heard of someone choosing to become homeless.

§

After I left the family's house, I walked back to the university and then into a university library, carrying only my small black shoulder bag. It was late March. I sat down at a desk alone. After about an hour, I walked from the library to a student lounge where I sat down in one of the comfortable couches. Not knowing what to do, I fell asleep. When I woke up, I had slept for most of the night in the building. I promptly left. No one seemed to have noticed.

The next morning, I went to the library again. I tried to read a school newspaper, but I could not focus. My mind was like a broken record thinking of nothing but what I had seen overseas and shutting out everything else. I was becoming hungry.

Later in the morning, about eleven, I realized I had not eaten in twenty-four hours. I still had no money and no ideas about where to get free food. I returned to the lounge where I had fallen asleep. But even as I sat there hungry, there was a burning passion inside me like a fire. I believed I was capable of doing something to help the poor overseas. I believed that I would someday do something great, and that my family and friends would see and be proud and amazed.

A few minutes after I returned to the lounge, I was met by an older Hispanic custodian who introduced herself as Carolyn. She asked me if I was all right. I must have looked hungry, because she gave me a large plastic container filled with chicken, rice and scrambled eggs. She did not seem to care who I was or why I was there, but only that I looked sick. She asked me no other questions. I cannot remember exactly what I told Carolyn that day about previously being a student, but she did not care about my explanations.

Carolyn later gave me food on several occasions during the following months. After seeing her a few times, I thought of asking Carolyn to let me go home with her. I think she would have let me. But I knew that if I stayed with Carolyn, I would have soon been expected to stand on my own two feet, to return to school or find a job. Since I resolved to not try working or going back to school, knowing I would fail, I never considered asking Carolyn for more help.

§

I spent the night in the lounge where I met Carolyn a couple of times. There was a restroom in the building that no one seemed to ever use, and I was able to wash up there late at night. But one evening, a police officer checked the lounge, and he told me it was an unsafe place to be at night.

Though I could no longer stay in the lounge during the nights, I found few students ever went there during the days. I would often stay for many hours. On weekends, I began sometimes staying there as many as six or eight hours at a time. I would think about my life and daydream. With the passing days, my desire to be alone grew even worse. Every day I started to spend at least a couple of hours alone thinking and staring into space. But whenever I encountered other people, I would become wide awake and behave normally.

During the next few months, I saw Carolyn now and then. She gave me homemade food and sometimes single dollar bills to get coffee or snacks from a machine.

§

In late March of 2003, I began spending my nights in a dormitory lounge that was a couple floors below the dormitory room I lived in during my freshman year. Since it had been years since I lived in the dormitory, the students there did not know me. When I began sleeping there, I was still using restrooms in the university area in the most hidden places, washing up at odd hours.

The resident assistant in the dormitory was friendly. I told him I was a student, as I still believed I had the rights of a student, but I gave few details. He invited me into his apartment by the lounge and gave me some snacks.

One night, I saw a flier advertising a dormitory party where there would be a movie and cake. When I arrived, I saw all of the students attending were eating the cake while watching a movie. But I could no longer stand to be around most people, especially groups of people, even if they had food and I was hungry. I was becoming antisocial. I attended the party, but after I ate some cake, I promptly left.

While I was leaving, I saw the students were wondering who I was and what I was doing. I felt guilty afterward, and I never attended another event like that again.

After I rested in the dormitory lounge for a few nights, the resident assistant told me that I could not stay there, and that I should go back to my apartment. He did not seem to know I had turned in my keys. It seemed no one knew I had chosen to move out.

When I was kicked out of the lounge, I considered spending some of my nights in a university library where I hoped to work online at night. I planned to write memoirs of what I had seen during my travels and email friends overseas. While I was a student, I never stayed up all night in the library, but many of my friends did regularly.

My first night in the library, I was surrounded by students studying hard, and I felt like a student again. I fell into a deep sleep on a comfortable padded library chair, and no one noticed. The next night, I spent some time online working on my nonprofit's website. Then, I slept in the library again.

§

I soon found that early in the night, after the university police had checked everyone's IDs, students in the library who dosed off late were usually ignored, and even welcomed. Prior to the arrival of the custodians, few students were around, and the library was full of leftover food. During my years as a student, I never noticed the leftover food before.

One night, I quickly and secretively walked around the library building to find some untouched sandwiches, coffees and other food that had been left. I thought it was odd to find so much food. Food was not even technically allowed in the library.

I started eating leftover food once in a while. I only looked for food occasionally, when I was certain no one was around. But after a few weeks, I began regularly looking for trashed leftover food, often scavenging at two or three o'clock every morning. It seemed that I always went unnoticed.

From the beginning of my time as a homeless person, I was determined to never go to a food bank, push a shopping cart, collect cans or garbage for money, or ask strangers for help. I hoped that while appearing to be a student, I could raise money for Africa.

While living in the library, I put up fliers at the university to recruit students to raise money for Africa. I found a few students who wanted to help. I saw them rarely and communicated with them over email. Once or twice that spring, I met with some interested students on the university campus. We talked about my goals. Most of them had no idea what my personal living situation was or that I had dropped out of college.

Because I had become homeless, I met much less often with international students. The huge international board meeting I had envisioned during 2002 never happened.

From late March onward, I made a huge, daily effort to hide my "homelessness." My small black shoulder bag appeared to be a stuffed computer case, though it was packed with changes of light clothing and not a laptop. I had good hygiene and tried to live and act like a student. I often wondered whether or not I was actually "homeless."

One afternoon in late March of 2003, near the beginning of my time as a homeless person, I was getting tired of washing the best I could in restrooms at odd hours. That day, I gave up, and I took a water bottle into a public restroom where I started carefully washing up in the stall. I thought I could hide and wash up unnoticed, even though there were other girls in the restroom. But I was wrong. Some girls called the police. When they came, a female officer told me I needed to "be more careful" and to clean up any water spill I might accidently cause. It was horribly embarrassing.

That day, one of the officers asked for my student ID. After she made a phone call, she found I had dropped out of the university, and she told me I was not a student. I was angry, thinking of my past good grades and research experience, and how hard I had worked. I thought of my goals and mission, and the money I was determined to send overseas. I thought of how, someday, the university would be proud of me.

Even after the humiliation, I still never considered entering a homeless shelter. I decided instead to be much more careful to wash up in restrooms when no one was around. I learned the times when various restrooms were not in use. I would quickly wash up in the early mornings or late at night. I found some restrooms were used so infrequently that I could wash my waist-long hair without being noticed. When I washed my hair, I worried every second that someone would walk in on me. But as the months went by, no one did, and I went unnoticed for over a year. When I washed my hair, I used hand soap. My hair always looked a little oily, but it was not yet bad enough to draw attention to me. I was occasionally meeting with students who did not seem to notice. I was meeting now and then with two professors who I had spoken with during the fall.

I was certain that my appearance and behavior appeared to be normal. One day, I met with a friend from the university who offered to help me file a complaint about the university police. We discussed what had happened on the day the girls in the bathroom had called the police. I believed I had been unfairly treated. Though it amounted to nothing, I remember just how sure I was that I was doing nothing wrong. I imagined filing complaints on the university police again later in life when I was rich and successful. If I had been thinking clearly, I would never have dreamed of trying to hold them accountable for their rudeness when I was acting so odd.

My life continued day after day, week after week, and then month after month as I inappropriately used restrooms, slept in libraries, ate leftover food and worked on my paperwork and website for my nonprofit. I felt no shame. I believed I was just like everyone else. I continued to believe anyone might readily mistake me for a part-time university graduate student, but that I was something better than that.

§

Though I was unable to study in fall of 2002, I figured out how to do the necessary paperwork for my nonprofit to become tax-exempt, with the help of some older friends. I had applied for tax-exempt status before I traveled to Thailand. In late March 2003, I received a letter informing me that the nonprofit had been granted tax-exempt status. I believed my goal of raising money was finally possible. I remembered the realities in Africa I had seen. I thought it would be easy to raise millions. But I had cut off everyone in my life who would have wanted to help me most.

I contacted more university friends, mostly Americans, who knew international humanitarian aid workers. I collected contact information and email addresses and wrote to them. I asked how much money they needed for their medical work and to buy medications to give the poor for free. I thought of how I was about to become rich. I spent hours alone thinking, daydreaming, and staring into space as I prepared for the money that I believed was about to come in.

I often wrote emails to international aid workers during the night when I could not sleep. It would reassure me that I had no place to stay the night for a good reason. One day, I wrote an email to a medical missionary in South America promising to send thousands of dollars to his charity. But as time went by, I kept telling him it was coming while I delayed, waiting for money to be raised. He finally wrote back, offended that I never sent the promised money.

I continued to believe I would someday be the one to provide funding for these groups. I was blind to my homelessness, delusional, and seriously beginning to lose weight.

CHAPTER FOURTEEN

The university library was designed to enable students to stay the night and study at anytime. I was living there, though too out of touch to know what I was doing. I was still somehow maintaining acceptable hygiene.

In spring of 2003, more than six months after our disagreement, the situation with my family had not changed. I still refused to speak with any of them. My hurt was as fresh as if I had disagreed with my parents a few days prior. My goals became my reason to live. When family and friends expressed disapproval of my passion, I could not tolerate hearing it from them. I do not know if it was the experience of Africa or simply because of my deteriorating mind, but I was unable to stand anyone's disapproval of my life choices. My parents continued to try to send me cards and packages, but I returned them or threw them away.

Continuing to look for food without being noticed was difficult. During April 2003, a month after losing my apartment, I began to look for small local parties (most of them around the university) and when they ended, I would go collect their unwanted leftover food. I continued to search for leftover food in the middle of the night. But in late spring of 2003, finding food left from parties and in other places was not enough. I was suffering from weight loss and hunger, and sleeping in the library was becoming miserable. I struggled to stay clean, and I always felt dirty underneath my clothes.

I continued to believe that if I were to maintain separation from my family and friends, I could not act like a homeless person. Months passed, and I never went to a homeless shelter, collected cans or begged. I did not want my parents, other relatives, or friends hearing that I had been seen on the streets or in a shelter and was obviously homeless. I feared that if I were living on the streets, my parents would try to use legal means to force me to come off the streets.

§

When I looked for leftover food, I often encountered a nice-looking young African man whose accent led me to believe he was from West Africa. I saw him frequently when I was secretly trying to find leftover food. I saw that he was also searching for food all over the place, just like me. Years later, I saw him at a church service where he was passing out hymnals, and I am almost certain that sighting at the church was a hallucination. I do not know whether the presence of this man in my life was completely real, a hallucination or sometimes a hallucination. I think my mind created another person in the same situation as me to comfort me.

In spring of 2003, I posted fliers again to recruit students to help me raise money for Africa. A young female student responded to one of the fliers that I posted. In late spring, I met her and talked with her about raising funds for building a new medical clinic in Nairobi. It meant everything to me. I described the medical clinic where I had volunteered and that I wanted to build a similar facility. She had connections with wealthy people.

As the academic semester was ending, the library was going to be closed during the nights in summer. I had been living in the library almost every night from March until early May. The first night the library was about to close, I sat alone at a library desk thinking. I was desperate for a place to live, or just to sleep. I believed in my heart that my lifestyle was morally right.

I planned to spend the first night the library was closed by hiding in a stairwell of one of the surrounding buildings. When I got to the building and walked up several floors, I found that the stairwell door to the building was not locked. The apartment building was partially vacated for the summer. In part of the building, all the apartments were open with the couches and bed mattresses still in place. The furniture was large and heavy, so there was nothing that could easily be stolen.

I stayed in the complex my first night of that summer, where I slept on a mattress. I experienced great comfort after having slept so many nights on the chairs in the libraries. I left the complex early the next morning.

I had wanted to spend just one night in one of the unlocked

apartments in the building, but no one seemed to notice me. I did it a second time, then the next night, and then the next. I suppose no one ever imagined that a person would actually enter the side entrance and stay the night. Though I was anxious at first that I would be discovered, I stayed in the empty apartments most of the summer without being noticed at all. When classes began, the library was open during the nights again.

When summer of 2003 was nearly over, my friend with the wealthy connections notified me that she had raised the thousands of dollars necessary to build the new medical clinic in Nairobi. The money came from foundations and individuals she knew well who were impressed by the building proposal I had put together. I immediately sent the money to the Kenyan foundation that was funding the building project. I received a canceled check from my nonprofit's bank account proving the money had been deposited in the right Nairobi bank account. I was thrilled.

Building a new clinic was what I had dreamed of doing while in Kenya, but the Kenyan foundation was slow to give me more updates. I became discouraged.

That summer, I wrote to the donors my friend had recruited. I thanked them and provided receipts for their tax-exempt donations. I planned to send them updates and pictures from Africa. I wish I had traveled to Kenya again about that time to witness the beginning of the building project. I regret not trying to visit Africa again at that time.

I did not know that I would not return to Africa again.

As summer ended, I continued to live out of my small black laptop case. It still looked new. I had three or four outfits that were planned carefully with light clothes and blouses. I could appear to have changed while wearing the same skirts. I decided to wear skirts and dresses all the time, and I looked more formal than the students. I felt as if I were above the students, smarter than they were, and more important.

In fall 2003, the students returned, and the university came alive again. As classes began, no one seemed to notice I had dropped out of school. I still spent countless hours in the library, usually working on my nonprofit's website. At night, I was invisible again while I showed staff my university ID and slept in corners of the library.

One day, while I was dosing off in a university lounge, someone stole my black bag. The bag contained my wallet, as well as all my carefully hidden clothing. I was irresponsible for not keeping copies of my identification and bank card. With my bag gone, I had no copies of my credit card numbers, contact information for my bank, or other personal identification.

I set off in search of my lost bag, and I found all of my things scattered at the end of the nearest hall, beside my empty bag. The thief apparently chose to leave my worthless things rather than take them. But he or she must not have looked through my things carefully, and I found my wallet untouched. I picked up my rejected belongings. I wondered if the thief had perhaps felt a surge of compassion after he or she saw I was not carrying a laptop. I became aware of my helplessness.

§

I began, again, to try to raise money to build or fund other clinics. Instead of closely tracking the building project in Nairobi, which I should have done, I focused on new projects. Purchasing medical supplies in Nigeria to give to the poor there for free seemed to be a good goal. That fall, I contacted David and Ruth in Nigeria. I hoped someday I might meet them again.

As I was spending every night in the library again that fall, I became a little smarter about where and when I was sleeping. I used computers that were only accessible to students with a university ID. I worked online at night. When I could not think of any more international friends to write late at night, I stayed awake by surfing the Internet. During the day, I located places in the university area where I could dose off.

That fall, I thought again of my past good grades, my research publications, and of my time as concertmaster of the university community orchestra. Even though I received C's my last semester, while planning my trip to Africa, I was a student then. I thought I still appeared to be a dedicated, nice, hard-working student.

I got to know some of the custodians who arrived in the library early in the mornings. I often visited Carolyn. I saw local police occasionally, and they smiled at me.

Though my experiences doing research had been some of the happiest times of my life, that fall, I never considered getting a job in research again. Sometimes I thought of how much I had enjoyed research, but I told myself doing research was below me. I believed I was the same person I had been in college, but I was not. I was in a mental fog that was only worsening, and I had become even less able to work or study.

Going to Thailand and Boston cost me thousands of dollars which I owed to two different credit card companies, but I was still certain somebody who believed in my cause would come into my life and pay them off. I felt excited about the person who I believed was coming, who would financially save my life.

A trip back to Kenya or Nigeria seemed too expensive and too emotionally draining. When I thought about returning to Africa, I imagined myself going with lots of money to give and visiting the new or nearly finished Nairobi clinic building. I continued to believe that my cause was divine, though I shared this with no one (except my parents and their friends in 2002, before we became estranged).

§

Though I was unable to visit David and Ruth in Africa, I wanted to hear more from them about the medical needs of the Nigerian poor. I suggested we meet in Europe, since it was a middle point between the United States and Nigeria. I never considered that I did not have enough money to fly to Europe.

David and Ruth responded to my email promptly and told me that they attended an annual conference in London in November, 2003. About a hundred students from all over Europe were to meet and discuss international politics. They said several political officials from Europe would be present, as well as other notable guests. They invited me to come. But David and Ruth thought Americans were rich. They were rich themselves. They had no idea that my financial situation was dire.

§

That fall, I met a new friend at the university. His name was Adam.

Adam was often in the library when I was. I saw him in passing all over campus. We eventually saw each other so many times that we smiled at each other, decided to introduce ourselves, and began to talk. We joked that we were destined to meet.

One night, Adam invited me to dinner across the street from campus and paid for everything. When he bought me dinner, costing about twenty dollars for both of us, I realized it was some of the only food that had been purchased for me in the last seven months. I thought of the great contrast to my freshman year at the university when I was living in the honors dormitory, and my parents bought me the meal plan. I remembered how, during my sophomore and junior years, I bought whatever groceries I wanted.

As we talked, I found out that Adam was an international student in the university's engineering program. He was knowledgeable of international politics, well-mannered, polite and handsome. He was dedicated to his studies, did not drink, and had high standards of moral integrity and a close-knit family. I admired him.

I talked for hours with Adam about my experience in Africa and my love of China. I explained to him that I raised money for the poor in Nairobi during the summer. He had great interest in the fundraising I had done and the money I hoped to raise for Africa and Thailand in the future. As I talked with Adam, I felt like I could do anything.

About the time I met Adam, I was staying briefly as a guest with a friend, a young female student, in her apartment. I did not want Adam to know that I had nowhere to stay. I lied to him, saying that I had a permanent place to live. I alluded to the place where I was briefly staying with my female friend.

After I got to know him better, I told Adam about my invitation to travel to London for three days. I told him that I wanted to meet people who could help me raise money and give me advice. I explained to him that I felt the opportunity to visit both Europeans and my African friends in London was worth the money it would cost to go. I told Adam I could not afford to go.

Soon after, Adam paid for us both to go to dinner again nearby the university. Over dinner, he told me he believed in me and in giving money to the poor. He said his family and friends in his home country also believed in giving money to causes like mine. That night, Adam wrote a check for the full cost of my trip, including airfare and conference fees.

§

As I prepared to go to London, I had certain needs, including getting some nicer clothing. I only owned the few outfits I was carefully storing in my black computer case. I wanted to look especially nice while I was traveling and meeting new people.

Even my closest friends seemed unaware I was homeless. One of my old university roommates from my sophomore year had brought my fliers to her mother who later donated money that I sent overseas. When I told her a little about my invitation to visit London and not having the funds to travel, she encouraged me. She was happy for me when the young man agreed to sponsor my trip, and I had purchased my tickets to London. I contacted her to ask if she had any nice clothing she could share with me, since we were about the same size, and she gave me a bag of beautiful clothes she no longer wanted. I reluctantly gave away everything that would not fit in my small black case. I wanted to keep all of the colorful and expensive used clothes, but I had no place to store them.

Through all of my preparations, I stuck to my resolution to never tell anyone I was homeless. In retrospect, I am sure that both Adam and my old roommate who gave me the clothing would have helped me escape from my homeless life if I asked. Instead, I was sleeping in the library and searching for food while I prepared to fly to England. And I was not aware that my dad was on his way to try to find me.

CHAPTER FIFTEEN

In October 2003, when I had not contacted my family for over a year, my dad made the long flight out west to try to find me and talk. To this day, I do not know how we happened to meet. The university area was huge, and I was usually busy inside the library and spent little time walking the campus. But one day, I ran into him near a library in the university area.

When I saw him from a distance, I did not know who he was, and was ready to say hello to a friend. But when I saw it was him, I became angry and ran away from him into one of the nearby buildings. I was desperate to have my relationship with my parents severed. I did not trust them, and I knew I could not work or go to school. I wondered if they might fight my fundraising efforts.

I hid from him for several minutes in one of the buildings. All I wanted was to avoid him. I wondered if he would find a way to prevent me from going to London or try to harm me in some other way.

After I hid from him for several minutes and was certain he would be gone, I went to the library and emailed my parents. I threatened legal action if they tried to contact me again. I told them I would call their friends and spread untrue rumors about them if they continued bothering me. I was afraid of them.

§

There were few people on my overnight flight to London. It was late November. I noticed most of the travelers were middle-aged men wearing suits. Many of them were spread over a few seats, sleeping. I was grateful for the free airline food since I did not have to scavenge. I wondered if anyone else on the plane was especially grateful for the free food.

The flight from the university area to London was nonstop. After I landed, I took a train to connect with several young people, mostly from Europe, who were waiting for a bus to the conference center. When I approached the group, I saw a tall, beautiful African woman who I knew as Ruth, my host from Lagos. Since I had lost so much weight and was wearing bright red lipstick, she did not recognize me at first. But after we met, Ruth and I talked as we excitedly traveled together on a bus to the conference center. I told Ruth about how I expected to be married soon, giving few details. I was thinking about the "savior" who I was still expecting to come.

Unfortunately, when Ruth and I arrived at the conference, I could barely focus. I cannot remember all the details of what happened because of my single-mindedness. I was walking around with arrogance, uninterested in the other people my age. I had become like a robot, set in one gear to raise money. I noticed there were no Chinese people in attendance, and I suggested that they invite Chinese people the following year. I made lots of other suggestions about how to improve their annual conference, though it was not my place. I talked on and on about fundraising to people who were not interested.

The conference was for Europeans only, and the few from Africa and America were special guests. But I forgot I was a special guest, and I should have been sensitive. I was rude and unable to relate properly to the people who invited me to the conference.

While in London, I began telling people my parents had recently died. The phrase was, to me, a half-truth. I believed I would never see my parents again. I felt the best description of this relationship was that both parties were as good as dead to each other. I told people they both were suddenly dead without giving any explanation or showing grief. I talked about having little money. I thought highly of myself. I forgot that in America, where I would soon return, I was homeless.

§

That weekend, despite my arrogant attitude and inability to concentrate, I did successfully speak with David and Ruth. They were happy for me that my friend and I raised money for the Nairobi clinic during the summer. They encouraged me to continue my efforts to send aid to Africa. They seemed interested in my nonprofit work. But I could have had a similar conversation with them over the phone.

Before I left London, some students, a Member of Parliament and I all stayed up late talking about the homeless epidemic in American cities. When I told the Member of Parliament about my international travels and the things I had seen overseas, he told me I should consider pursuing a career in politics. I thought about the "savior" I was still expecting to come into my life and give my charity lots of money and marry me. I thought that perhaps my future husband, the "savior," would have a career in politics. That night, I told the Member of Parliament I wanted to marry a politician.

During the conference, I spent a lot of time thinking about my life. I began to realize that, despite my homelessness, I was happy with my life. Knowing that miracles would happen and money would come was exhilarating. I constantly and unconditionally believed in my cause while I enjoyed working toward it with great expectations.

By the end of 2003, I had fallen more deeply into a very thick mental cloud. I knew it was happening. I simply trusted in God that my mental sharpness would someday return. I reasoned there was nothing else I could do. I believed a miracle was my only hope.

§

While in England, my homelessness was invisible, except for one incident. Before I flew back to America from London, I was about fifteen pounds short on train fare to go from the conference center back to the airport. It was a small amount, but there was no bank account I could draw funds from. (I had maxed out my credit cards about a year before, on my Thailand trip). When I told a couple of people I lacked about fifteen pounds, they welcomed me to go with them to a local ATM. They seemed to have no idea I was actually asking them for money.

When David and Ruth heard I needed money, though I do not remember telling them I needed it, they immediately gave me twenty pounds without asking any questions. I hoped they would give me the benefit of the doubt and overlook the inconsistency of lacking personal money while trying to raise money. I hoped they thought I had simply forgotten to withdraw money at the ATM.

Before I left the conference, there were a few people who commented that I was unusually thin and looked ill, but I tried to explain it was "normal" for me. Since I was well-spoken, dressed nicely, and generally appeared normal, I believe my paleness and weight loss were mostly overlooked. My new European friends recommended I stay in the country and travel. I simply told them I had to leave.

I returned to the university area after my long flight back from London. On my return, all I wanted was to wash my hair. I snuck into a bathroom where I knew there was almost never anyone. I locked the door and washed myself and my long hair. My three day trip was over, and I felt like I was home.

I had severe jet lag upon my return. I checked a classroom that was usually locked, but I found it open, and I lay down on the carpet in the front by the whiteboard. I slept for many hours on the carpet.

After my trip to London, I felt that I was looking on life with a better international perspective. I thought a lot about how the Member of Parliament told me I should consider a career in politics. I felt the trip had been a success. I believed the university should have been grateful that I was still around, though I had dropped out before graduation.

When I returned from England, it was near the end of November. Before the Christmas holiday of 2003, some old friends emailed me to invite me to attend a Chinese Christmas celebration. I had not seen those friends in years. Since I had gone to China briefly in January of 2002 and January of 2003, and knew some phrases in Chinese, I was excited to go to the party. I showed up at the party wearing my nicest long skirt. As always, I was carrying my computer case stuffed with light clothing, and was careful never to open the case.

While at the party, I met a Chinese girl, a friend who I had not seen in months. She came up to me, dropped her jaw, and said that she could barely recognize me. She asked if I had been ill, as I had lost so much weight. I tried to make light of her comments and enjoy the rest of the time at the party. I have been thin my whole life. Though I did not know my weight at that time, I estimate I had lost ten or fifteen pounds in the past year. Searching for food was not working out.

§

During Christmas of 2003, the library where I spent most of my time was closed, but there were others open in the area. Throughout the holiday, I found myself missing friends and family. I was not angry with them, but continued seeing them as heartless. I spent Christmas Day writing about Africa for many hours in a computer laboratory. It helped me shut out the pain of having lost all of my family and nearly all my friends. I wanted to contact some students who supported my nonprofit and talk to them, but it was difficult to explain why I was not beginning a Ph.D. I would have been embarrassed and ashamed if they discovered I did not finish my bachelor's degree. Throughout the following years, it would always seem that no one ever noticed I did not graduate.

After visiting London, I had lots of ideas. But to raise more money, I began to see I needed a college degree or a miracle, or probably both.

§

During the holiday break, I was alone and lonely, but since the campus was deserted, it was easy to find empty restrooms to wash up in. There was little food to be collected, but I did find some. I found a small, empty auditorium in the university area where I could spend the night sleeping on a carpet by an exit. I laid my head against my black computer case and a colorful scarf, and I was ready to hurry out through the exit, unseen, if anyone came in. Since I had spent nine months sleeping on uncomfortable chairs or mattresses, I fell into a deep sleep on the carpet in seconds.

During the night in the empty auditorium, I had a dream where I saw evil spirits, and I saw God was fighting for my cause. The dream thrilled and excited me. After the dream, I no longer felt lonely. My deteriorating mind was trying to make sense of the bizarre life I had chosen.

By the end of the Christmas season, I finished putting together my document describing my international experiences. Most of it had been written on Christmas Day. But though I enjoyed writing, I was in denial. To me, the people in Africa were not poor, not suffering, and not gravely in need. I saw the beauty of the people, their culture and their land.

When the Christmas season ended, I emailed my manuscript to many people, but most of them did not care to respond. Some who wrote back were annoyed by my persistence. Others read parts of it and found my thinking confused and my opinions ridiculous.

After the Christmas holiday, my favorite library reopened. I was back in the library nearly every night.

By January 2004, I was even more underweight. I was losing my daily battle to secretly find food from parties or in the libraries. My mind was getting more fuzzy. I was still incapable of studying or working even the easiest job, so I never considered working or studying. I remembered that, in 2002, my best efforts in school had produced failing grades, and by 2004, my mind had clouded much more.

I was beginning to feel like my life was a videogame that I had to somehow escape. By not working or going to school, I escaped the videogame. Perhaps through isolation, I felt a sense of relief. If I had been offered a hundred thousand dollars a year in 2004 to work an easy job, I would have refused it. I wanted instead to feel detached from reality. Almost no amount of money would have convinced me to join the work force. Even today, having a job or attending classes would make me feel like I was in a huge trap, or a frightening jail cell.

Despite the fog in my mind, I found I was still able to memorize things such as vocabulary words. I could read, though I was unable to study complicated material like biology.

In early 2004, I stopped making much effort to fundraise.

CHAPTER SIXTEEN

Adam was preparing to return to his home country after Christmas and was less busy. In January 2004, he introduced me to some new people. Through him, I met students from Africa, China and the Middle East. Some of the people I met would occasionally invite me to dinners. I fought to maintain good hygiene, and, somehow, I succeeded.

I especially loved spending time with one of the new people I met through Adam, a Chinese scientist named Joshua. Joshua was generous, and I soon began going out with him often. He always paid for my dinner whenever we ate together, and he never asked for anything in return.

As I got to know Joshua better, I told him I was not enrolled in classes. When he asked where I lived, I lied, saying that I was living in one place or another. I told Joshua I had different "roommates," referring to friends I hardly knew. Sometimes I would stay with university friends for a few days at a time, but I would tell him I was a guest at their homes indefinitely. It was what I told everyone who asked. I remembered being treated like garbage in Boston when I told the airport chaplain I had no place to stay.

My inability to work or study felt like a personal problem. I never considered telling Joshua my mind was in a thick cloud.

Joshua never asked for details about where I lived or what exactly my address was. But after a few weeks, I did find the courage to admit to him that I had no permanent home. He did not seem surprised, as he must have suspected it. But when I told Joshua the truth, he was concerned.

§

As I got to know Joshua better, I mentioned several times that I had no interest in dating or marrying anyone at that time in my life. But I began seeing Joshua almost every day. I talked often about my experience in Africa. I had never had a boyfriend before, and did not want to begin dating in my homelessness. But I was mentally dull enough to believe he would accept my repeated statements that I did not yet want to marry or date. I did not realize that he was seriously interested in having a relationship with me.

Over the years, there were many young Christian men who were college students who took me out to dinner or to events or parties without seeking to date me. This included the man who paid to have my airline ticket changed in Boston. He paid for the change without asking any questions or asking for anything in return. I thought that my relationship with Joshua would be the same.

I had always been fascinated by Chinese culture, and I loved Joshua's stories, seeing pictures of his family, and hearing about his work in engineering. But as a child, I was taught that successful marriages came from two mature and well-adjusted people coming together. My nonprofit had not yet succeeded, and I was unable to work a job. I waited for the millions of dollars I believed were coming, and for the "savior."

§

As hard as I tried to hide it, when I got to know Joshua better, he learned I was short on food. One day, he expressed his firm belief in me and in what I wanted to do for Africa. He told me that his family was interested in helping me out financially, but only me personally. He explained that the money was for me and not for my charity work. Joshua knew that, had he let me, I would have immediately either sent the money to Africa or used the money to travel to the new Nairobi clinic.

During the next few weeks of February 2004, Joshua provided some limited funding for me to buy food. The cheapest thing I could find was pizza at a local cafeteria, and I went there often. Joshua took me out to lunch and dinner several more times. That February, I began to gain my weight back. All of the new friends I met through Adam were surprised at how much healthier I looked.

Joshua was the only person that knew I had no permanent place to live. None of the other friends I made that winter sought to know the exact details of my living situation. My university ID was still active, and I was able to carry on intelligent conversations like the students, so most of my friends just assumed I had a place to live. I would sometimes allude to my published research papers available on the Internet, hoping no one who saw my publications would ever wonder if I might be homeless. There were people I met who saw me wearing the same clothes many days and probably did not believe I was the same "Bethany Yeiser" who had authored three publications in science.

Despite my failing mind, I occasionally met with university students interested in my organization. I explained that we had raised money and sent it to Nairobi. I was excited that the organization was tax-exempt and official. But as it turns out, I never raised much more money.

§

Joshua saw that all I cared about was the nonprofit. He was too polite to tell me my dreams were unrealistic, or that I should give up. But he recognized that I was in a miserable situation, sleeping in different places on different nights, and not having enough food.

Joshua realized that since I was not taking classes, I was free to move. He suggested I should, hoping to provide a safer place for me to stay with good people. That February, he offered to fly me to New Mexico to stay with Chinese-American friends of his family.

The emerging changes in my personality at that time were not yet bad enough to be noticed by friends. I was still occasionally speaking about my travels with various professors on campus, as well as with students and other people. I was not hallucinating, or at least not very much. But although I could have recalled a thousand details about my childhood, it was as if the details of my past life belonged to another person.

The trip to New Mexico was paid for in full by my Chinese friend's family. I was excited to meet them. Once again, I left my homeless life in the university area to go on another trip.

§

When my flight to New Mexico landed, I met my host family there and saw they were friendly, kind and smart people. I was given a comfortable bedroom suite with its own bathroom in their home. I got together with the family for all of my meals, which included lots of delicious, home-cooked Chinese food. Like many of my Chinese friends, they were surprised I could use chopsticks well. I was thankful for having a place to stay, and to be around a family again. Sleeping in a bed was wonderful.

I was happy with my host family for a few days. But by my fourth or fifth day there, I changed. I became agitated all the time, and I became unhappy and temperamental. I was extremely sensitive, though there was no real reason why. I missed Joshua, and I was bored. I found I missed the exhilaration of having to look for food, and the deceptive homeless life I lived near the university. I began to miss never knowing for sure where I would be staying the night.

After the first few days in the comfortable and beautiful home, I became antisocial. I went on their computer in a bedroom and continued to write about my travels, working on the document I began during Christmas. I spent most of my time alone in the bedroom writing. Every minute I could, I avoided the family. After a few days, I could not stand living in a normal home again.

At first, Joshua's Chinese-American friends did not seem to notice, but after a few days, they saw I was unhappy. They were especially sensitive, and asked almost nothing, since I was offended by any mention of school and any questions about my parents. They never encouraged me to work and did not pressure me to return to school. They were excited to hear about Africa when I talked about it. They also had a large network of international friends from many countries. I loved meeting more international people.

Even after I had changed and become irritable, my host family gave me no pressure to return to the west. I was welcome to stay with them indefinitely, and it seemed they cared deeply about me.

I wanted to stay in the home of my host family with the benefits of having food, my own bathroom and so many new friends. But even after just a few days, regular life was too boring for me. I loved Chinese culture, but in 2004, I could not stand living with a normal American family, not even one from China.

Years later, after I had been jailed for trespassing on the campus when I was homeless, I would still not ask to return to New Mexico to live with the Chinese-American family in their home.

§

After my week with the family, I told them I was ready to leave and return out west. They were perplexed, but in kindness, they overlooked my odd behavior and seemed to genuinely want me to stay.

I thanked them for their kindness but affirmed I needed to go.

At the end of the trip, the family took me to the airport, and as I was leaving, they gave me a few hundred dollars in cash. I was so touched by their generosity. But upon my return out west, I lost touch with them.

On my return, I saw Joshua. He was confused why I chose not to stay with his friends, but he did not ask many questions. He welcomed me back. I resumed spending my nights in the library. I continued to try to maintain good enough hygiene and appearance to meet new people and was successful.

§

As I spent more time with Joshua, I tried again to make it clear that I was not interested in a dating relationship. I still had no intention of marrying while I was so helpless, and while my "invisible" situation was so bizarre. I behaved as though I really did not know I was any different than anyone else, but I was somehow aware of my homeless situation.

Joshua eventually asked me about my debt, including my credit card debt. I remembered paying for my travels to Thailand on my credit cards, and how I had withdrawn cash from my credit cards, deposited it and sent it to clinics overseas. I owed credit card companies thousands of dollars.

Throughout the years, I never mentioned to anyone that I paid for my flight to Thailand using a credit card, and that I sent clinics overseas cash I withdrew from credit cards. Joshua never asked about what I had charged on my credit cards. I believed in my heart that my decision to travel to Southeast Asia in fall 2002 had been right, but I knew that I could appear unstable to other people. I imagined a mother maxing out her credit cards to pay hospital bills for her gravely ill child.

I also had other debt. I took out a large loan to pay for the classes I never attended in 2002-2003 when my best academic efforts were producing F's. I had much smaller loans I took to help pay for college from 1999 until 2002.

In March 2004, I admitted to Joshua that I had accrued credit card debt, and he told me he was interested in helping me pay it off. Since I had no money, I threw away bank statements that asked for repayment without even looking at them. Though I was in great need and it was not true, I assured Joshua that I did not need his financial help.

One day, Joshua asked for statements of what I owed to the two credit card companies. I gave him the statements, but never imagined he would contribute significantly. A few days later, I received an email that I should call one of the credit card companies in order to be certain my bill was paid off. When I called the credit card company, they told me my balance was zero. I was speechless. Later, I thanked Joshua, hoping I could repay him someday.

§

During March 2004, I thought about the year that had passed since I lost my apartment. From March 2003 to March 2004, I became homeless, sent funding to Nairobi, traveled to England and to New Mexico, and Joshua had paid off thousands of dollars of my debt. As the one-year anniversary of losing my apartment arrived, I found many events of the past year unbelievable.

I had no plans to travel again in 2004. When I contemplated my life, I felt certain that I was supposed to stay, remaining just as I was, even if it were for years. I still fervently believed the "savior" was coming, and I wanted to keep waiting for him. I did not see the absurdity of my decision to just sit in homelessness and do nothing. But since I could not work or study normally, there was nothing else to do.

As I began a second year as a homeless person, I found that fundraising was no longer possible. I viewed the thousands of dollars I had raised and sent overseas as amazing in itself.

§

In March 2004, I had more time on my hands, and I began using the Internet to teach myself the Hebrew alphabet and fifty of the most basic words in the ancient language. Though I still could not study biology, basic memorization of vocabulary words was possible. Just as I had wanted to study Biblical languages as a child (I had studied some Biblical Greek in high school), studying Hebrew delighted me.

I was in a daily routine where I would spend hours on a

computer working on my website, emailing international friends and studying Hebrew. Every day, when I finished working online and studying, Joshua would pick me up in his old car. We went out to eat at many places, often on the university campus. He always paid for everything. We talked about China. Joshua was extremely conservative, and he never even shook my hand, but our friendship was wonderful.

One day in March 2004, Joshua invited me to dinner at a fancy Japanese restaurant near the university. He told me that night that his family would be delighted if I would join him on his upcoming business trip to Taiwan to stay with them there. I told Joshua again that I could not have a serious boyfriend, and he assured me that he was not seeking to date me. Joshua said I was a good friend of his family. I was thrilled to accept Joshua's invitation to join him on his trip to Taiwan.

Joshua was not sure how long we would be in Taiwan, but estimated it would be a month. Before I went to Taiwan, I took the cash I had saved from my New Mexico trip and deposited it in the bank. I knew that if I encountered some emergency while in Southeast Asia, I had enough money to immediately fly back to America.

I could not believe I was getting to travel to Southeast Asia again.

CHAPTER SEVENTEEN

I left for Taiwan with Joshua in spring of 2004. After we landed in Taipei, we traveled to a small apartment in the heart of the city where his family lived.

While in Taiwan, there was an election which many Taiwanese people believed had been altered to select the candidate who did not really win. Because they believed the election was corrupt, half a million people took to the streets of Taipei. The protest occurred right after Joshua and I arrived in the country. Joshua, his mother, and I walked along with the mass of angry Taiwanese citizens out of curiosity. To restrict the movement of mobs, barbed wire was everywhere. Though police were on every corner, the three of us felt unsafe. I wondered if many people in America were closely following the disputed Taiwanese election.

After the rioting ended, Joshua, his mother and I enjoyed living in the city. We walked the streets, ate at restaurants, visited parks, and traveled to the mountains. I quickly came to love his family. Joshua spent time meeting Taiwanese scientists and discussing his research, which was the main objective of the trip.

While in Taiwan, I often thought of my situation back in America. My feelings were mixed. Sometimes I thought about Danielle, the young woman I helped visit Nairobi in 2002, and our friendship after she returned from Africa. Since Danielle understood what I had seen in Africa, I wondered if I could contact her and look for a job through her friends. I wondered if I could perhaps teach violin again, which I used to love. But when I tried to be honest with myself, I was torn between doing the logical right thing (getting some sort of a job) and following a mission and a dream that might be unrealistic. I thought of my successful Hebrew studies, and I told myself I could study biology again.

But something deep inside of me knew that choosing the logical action was impossible. In the past two years I had become more mentally foggy. I knew I could not work a job. Almost no salary was worth the feelings of being in touch with reality again. I knew my homelessness was bizarre, but life in a home like my Chinese-American family's home was too boring for me. I saw that in America, I preferred my homeless life.

I thought of the "savior." I believed that if I worked again and studied in school, the "savior" would not be interested in helping that kind of a normal person, and would never come to me. As for my real family, my Chinese host family in New Mexico, and the family of my Chinese friend, I never considered that any of them might be the "savior." I expected the "savior" had a law degree or was a politician.

After a few weeks in Taiwan, I had no desire to go back to America. I do not know why I was so happy in Taiwan and able to behave normally there, but unable to live with the Chinese-American family in New Mexico. I think it was because the exhilaration of encountering the new culture in Taiwan was as stimulating as my homeless life in America. As I quickly came to love Joshua's family, I focused on my present situation and context. With every passing week, I stopped longing as much for the "savior," and I thought less and less about raising millions of dollars. I felt that my mind was clearing, and it was clearer than it had been for years.

§

Even after a few weeks in Taiwan, I never spent time with Joshua in a private place, as just the two of us. We had no intimate relationship beyond our friendship. But on the trip, I was blind to his intentions and was too accepting of Joshua and his family's generosity. I felt like he and his parents were my family, and that my short explanation that I could not date was enough. I was used to American traditions where dating people spend time together alone and hug or kiss, but we never touched each other. He was so conservative that he never gave me a hug or a kiss on the cheek. Joshua and I had never spent even a minute discussing the future. But after three weeks in Taiwan, Joshua asked me to marry him.

When he asked me to marry him, I felt like I had just met him and did not know who he was. Though I felt terrible to refuse, I could not accept Joshua's proposal. I thought he was my friend, my supporter, and someone who believed in me, but not a boyfriend. I felt we had never shared a deep love. I told Joshua again I was not ready to marry anyone at that time. When I refused Joshua, he did not seem very upset.

After rejecting Joshua's marriage proposal, I told him I loved life in Taiwan, and that I wanted to stay in Taiwan, where I was thriving, for as long as possible. But after I said no to his proposal, he was ready for us both to return to America, and to the university.

Joshua and I left for the United States on a beautiful April morning, travelling on a bus to the airport with his mom. When we got off the bus, I was saddened that I might not see her again. I hugged her and cried.

After my return to America, I discovered that someone had paid off a few thousand more dollars of my personal debt, the remainder of what I owed on my credit cards. I am sure it was Joshua or his family.

§

Since I was not marrying, I found it necessary to not accept any more of Joshua's financial support. I felt it would be very wrong to take his money after rejecting his proposal, and I clung to my integrity. But he had been so helpful buying me food. I was grateful that I had regained my healthy weight, and I could not stand to lose the weight again.

On my return from Taiwan, I almost never carried any money, though there was some money in the bank that I never touched, which was deposited before I visited Taiwan. When I was hungry, waiting for parties to leave food and for everyone to be gone was not satisfactory. Sometimes, though not often, people saw me looking for food. I no longer cared. My mind had become broken. I began to do whatever it took to find leftover food. I began to live on leftover garbage just as I had been doing before I met Joshua.

Not seeing Joshua again also meant that I would not go to dinner or lunches with his group of friends, and I missed that terribly.

§

When the university's spring semester of 2004 was ending, I realized that the money I was given in New Mexico plus the money from Joshua for my personal needs meant I had enough to travel again. After ending my relationship with Joshua, I never considered spending the money on food or on myself. I was no longer accountable to him for what I spent, so I decided to spend the money on my charity.

Some of the Africans I met at the conference in London in 2003 had connections to indigenous clinics in Rwanda and Uganda. I wanted to learn more about the clinics and talk with the person who was running them. Since I was able to afford it, I decided to go to England again and collect information about more African charities.

I did not ask any of the few friends who were technically part of my organization to join me on my second trip to England, which was a mistake. That May, 2004, I left the libraries and the computer laboratories to travel to London again, alone.

CHAPTER EIGHTEEN

In May 2004, I went to visit a Ugandan charity director who lived in London. He traveled back and forth between Africa and London, sending money and support to two charities, one in Uganda, and the other in Rwanda. Both charities focused on feeding and providing basic needs for children. They had little financial support. The irony that I was working to feed starving children while I was nearly starving myself did not register with me.

The Ugandan man hosted me in a small house in a London suburb where he lived with other African nationals. Naïve, I could have easily been abused by the men living at the house. But I quickly came to trust them, and I felt safe.

During the week, while living in his home, I spoke with the Ugandan man about his work. Over simple dinners, and while spending time walking with him over his cobblestone suburb, he told me about his passion to care for forgotten children. He showed me videos of strikingly beautiful Ugandan toddlers and older children. I should have copied the videos and shown them to Americans. With these videos, I am sure I could have easily raised money in America, if I had a clear mind.

While in London, I visited my friend's church, filled with black Africans who lived in London. I joined them as they sang and danced late into the night.

As I left England for the second time, I gave my Ugandan friend a small check that came from the limited money I had remaining, leaving me about one dollar in my bank account. I was confident I would send his charities much more money in the future, though to this day, I have not yet sent them any more money.

When summer 2004 arrived, the library was closed for the nights again. I spent every night in the vacant apartment complex again, exactly as I had the year prior. Every morning, after I spent the night, I left the building early. Most days, I found comfort in watching the pink sunrise.

That summer, I usually entered the library at seven A.M., when it opened. I checked my email and began studying Hebrew. During the days, I rested in lounges in the university area, went for walks, and occasionally met with my few friends who were students. I did not usually see anyone I knew.

I continued to scavenge for food during the entire summer, but was more careful to do it secretly. I learned where to go to find the best food, often anxiously waiting for parties I saw to be over. Finding food was easier during the summers.

I thought of my parents occasionally. Though I was still sure I would never see them again, I thought they would someday see me on national news as a celebrity and be proud of me.

I slowly realized that I loved my life. It was somehow similar to how I felt living in Africa. The belief that someday I would make a difference in the world was real to me and filled me with excitement. Though I was not making sense, I was often happy.

By the end of the summer, 2004, I began reading some of the easier Hebrew Bible passages.

§

When fall came, I had been homeless for eighteen months, and I realized I had slept in the library too much. I was no longer invisible. I tried working in computer laboratories in the university area late at night instead of staying in the library. I hoped to blend in with the students. I soon made friends from among the students who regularly spent all night studying in the laboratories.

I do not remember that fall well, but I often stayed awake during the nights by studying Hebrew and surfing the Internet. I regularly fell asleep in the early hours of the morning with my forehead resting on the desks. The days began to blend together. While I was awake, studying something, anything, made me happy.

§

In late 2004, only a couple of friends from my university years, before I went to Africa, remained. The one and only remaining friend from my old church was Scott, the same man who drove me to the airport to fly to Boston in 2003. From 2003 until 2006, Scott would occasionally meet me in the campus area and buy me lunch. He always asked for more details about what I was doing. I told Scott I was sending money to Africa and studying Hebrew.

Scott never asked questions about my personal situation. I felt comforted to know that he had no interest in dating me, like other close male friends I made at my church years prior. Scott seemed to feel compassion for my changed situation, and he wanted to help.

On one occasion, years into my homelessness, I badly needed to buy some new shoes and clothing. I decided to contact Scott and ask if he would consider giving me some money. As soon as he received my email, Scott met me and took me to an ATM where he withdrew a hundred dollars and handed it to me. Scott said he remembered the times, years before, when I invited him over to my apartment for parties and dinners.

I had one other friend at the time who was a former university roommate. She had given me clothing for my trip to London, and her mother had donated money for me to send overseas. When my friend visited the university area, she occasionally treated me to ice cream or lunch. Sometimes she asked where I was living, but when I alluded to a building in the university area and lied to her that it was where I lived, it satisfied her. It satisfied everyone. I used to have as much money as she did, and she was perplexed that my situation had changed, and that I had lost everything.

§

In the fall of 2004, I abused my privileges at the university more than ever. When meeting friends at the library, or occasionally at parties, I continued to tell them I was a part-time graduate student. I invited them to view my three research articles on the Internet, published in 2002 and 2003. I still had my university ID at that time. I continued to study Hebrew and surf the Internet in a computer laboratory every night. When I occasionally attended social gatherings, few people asked questions.

I was still deluded to believe I had all the rights and privileges of a student. I imagined that, someday, the university would be proud of my success in Africa, and I became even more confident that this would happen. I was certain I was welcome at the university forever, and did not see that I did not belong there anymore. Some students I met asked why I had so few outfits, but I did not care.

Later that year, I made friends with a young woman from Saudi Arabia whose husband was a student, and she gave me a beautiful green dress. It appeared to be made in India or the Middle East. It fell to my ankles, and was lined with ribbons of blue, red and gold. The green dress fit my figure perfectly, as though it were made for me. After my friend gave me the green dress, I sometimes wore it many days in a row. I loved the dress.

I was unaware that the unusual dress was beginning to draw attention to me. Today, I wonder how much I began to stand out while walking the campus and wearing the green dress.

A few times, university police caught me resting in a lounge where only current students were allowed to be at night.

Over a period of two and a half years, when I was caught resting in lounges, I showed the police my university ID. At first, when the night police saw me there, they simply asked me to leave. Sometimes they made comments that I was behaving irresponsibly by being in the lounges at night, which was painful, but it did not happen often. The police began growing tired of seeing me, a former student who was not enrolled in classes, during the nights.

One night I was caught sleeping in a small student lounge in a tall campus building. That night the police not only wanted to see my ID, but asked me a series of questions. These included my mother's maiden name, when I began classes at the university, my birthday, and my major, all of which I knew how to answer. The officers seemed perplexed that I knew all the answers to their questions. They did not see that though I had the same body, I had a broken mind, and I had changed into a different individual.

Finally, it was simply a matter of being caught too many times, over too many months. Around three o'clock one morning, police confiscated my university ID.

A few hours later, when the police station opened, I went there to demand that my ID be returned. An older policeman invited me into his small office in the university police station. I looked over the newspaper clippings and awards in his office while I waited to speak with him.

The older policeman treated me with dignity, but seemed

confused by what had happened. I think he was surprised that I was acting so strange during the nights, and yet, I could speak confidently and intelligently with him, unlike a homeless person. I discussed my past high grades at the university and the research I used to do.

At first, the officer seemed to agree with me that I should have my ID back. After our meeting, I walked with him to another university building where we met with a student advisor. She asked me if I was attending any classes without paying for them, and I told her I was not.

Together, the policeman and the advisor decided they would keep my ID. Soon after, I discovered that my university email account had been deactivated.

§

Years passed before I was ever seen washing my hair, but I was eventually caught in a public restroom right after I washed my hair, and it was still wet. The police told me that day I should never be on the university campus again. But with my research experience at the university and former standing as a student, I was certain they were mistaken. That morning was the exception, as no one ever seemed to notice. I wondered why they cared I had wet hair.

I thought it was my legal right to ignore the officers. And even though the officers told me that I was never to return to the university, I knew that the university was open to the public. I thought the university had no right to deny me the privileges of the general community. I thought I was acting normally.

I wish the encounters with police had made me aware of my homelessness, and that the experience of being caught led me to find a place to live, such as a homeless shelter. But the encounters with police did not lead me to change anything.

CHAPTER NINETEEN

I spent Christmas Eve and Christmas Day of 2004 sleeping on the same front carpet of the same auditorium where I had slept the year before. I do not remember Christmas 2004 well, but I remember always being alone on the holidays.

After Christmas, I continued to study Hebrew every day. As March 2005 approached, the end of my second year homeless was almost over. It was two years since I had lost my university apartment.

In spring 2005, I attended a party for international students and Americans who were interested in meeting international students. The party was hosted by the same Caucasian couple who had invited me to a Christmas party in 2003. Since I had been in mainland China for ten days in 2002, Hong Kong for a week in 2003, and Taiwan for a month in 2004, I especially enjoyed meeting Chinese students. At the party, I wore my green dress. I tried my best to blend in with students and volunteers.

That night, I met a Chinese couple who had recently come to the United States. I found them to be kind and intelligent people. When I mentioned that I had been to China, spoke a few words and phrases in Chinese, and explained that I wanted to study more Chinese someday, they suggested I begin studying immediately. The couple offered me free lessons in exchange for help with English.

In April, I met weekly with the Chinese couple to learn Chinese tones and basic words. The couple taught me how to say things like "Hello, how are you," "It is raining," and "I study Chinese." I am grateful that during that confusing time of my life, I was able to do something productive.

While with the couple, I was careful to have good hygiene, wear different combinations of clothing from my shoulder bag, and do everything in my power to appear to be a student. I am certain the Chinese couple had no idea I was homeless or different from the university students. The Chinese couple was interested in my research from years before, and they asked lots of questions. I still loved speaking about my research, though I could not work. They invited me to their home occasionally, where they served me delicious, authentic Chinese dinners. I wish I could have brought them food.

There was only one incident when my secret homeless life may have become apparent to the Chinese couple. One night after our meeting, and after I said goodbye to them, I went and hid in a bathroom nearby that had a couch. No one ever seemed to enter the bathroom at night. But that night, the Chinese woman entered the bathroom and saw me sleeping on the couch. She was surprised at first, and then acted as if it were a coincidence and normal. I left immediately.

The following week, we resumed my Chinese lessons, as usual. The couple probably thought it was rude to ask about finding me in the bathroom late at night. They never mentioned it.

When summer came, I was becoming more antisocial, though I did not know it. I noticed in the early summer of 2005 that the Chinese man stopped inviting his wife to our sessions. I felt awkward about it, and I did not want to make him like me too much. I still do not know if I did it because he was really a bit too interested in me, or because I was acting strangely. But that summer, I made the decision to stop Chinese lessons.

§

During that summer, I used a first-year college textbook to start learning the most basic Chinese characters on my own. I found myself living a quiet and happy life while I was engrossed in learning the complex, ancient and beautiful written language. During the nights, I hid in the same vacant apartment complex as before. Like the previous two summers, no one noticed me there.

During fall 2005, I completely stopped staying at the university libraries and computer laboratories. I had already been warned by police to never be on the campus again, but I believed that the officers who noticed me washing my hair had no authority to kick me off the campus, so I freely spent time on other parts of the campus.

I was exhausted, and I could not study anymore. Instead, I found a few new places where I could sleep, mostly in bathrooms no one seemed to use. I spent about thirty nights sleeping in a certain rarely-used bathroom on the ceramic tile floor. I was so tired that I always fell asleep there in seconds. Every morning, I would leave the restroom before anyone arrived, often at three or four A.M. When I left every day, I went and sat in various places outside near local apartment complexes where I would hide, dose off, and lightly sleep in the early morning hours.

Some of the best places I found to hide and rest were on porches of large apartment complexes. I was never noticed in any of these places. I would leave the grounds of the apartments about sunrise. I also spent a few nights sleeping on the concrete floor of a stairwell. No one noticed me.

I thought of myself as a good student of languages, since I studied both Hebrew and Chinese, and I never thought of myself as a homeless woman. I rarely thought about how much I used to love working in the biochemistry laboratories. There were times the thought that I was homeless plagued my mind. I wondered if I really was both a "normal" and a "homeless" person at the same time.

When November 2005 arrived, I was having trouble sleeping well. Sleeping every night in the public bathroom or the concrete floor in the stairwell was not working out because I was never able to sleep deeply. I started developing an eye infection, but I kept trying to sleep in the vacant restroom on the floor anyway. Since I was unnoticed, I continued it. I did not know what else to do.

§

Christmas 2005 was unlike the prior two Christmases I had spent in libraries. The only safe place I could find to stay was a seldom-used bathroom. The building with the restroom was locked from right before Christmas until after the holiday, and I would not have been able to get back in if I left. Before the holiday, I put together a collection of food for three days. I stayed in the building for all three days, spending most of the time catatonic in the same restroom.

The building where I was hiding was many stories high. On the morning of Christmas Day, I went many floors up to look out a window. Over that Christmas, it rained a lot. I was glad to be somewhere, anywhere, inside.

There was still a motivation and a burning zeal inside of me to continue waiting for the "savior," even when it hurt to be alone.

§

On New Year's Day of 2006, I emerged from the restroom. When I exited the building, I saw there were few people in the university area, but as I walked around, I saw small gatherings. I was especially hungry. As I checked in places where I usually found food, I became discouraged. Public safety officers were driving around the campus on holidays. I hated walking alone all over the university area while trying to keep my search for food a secret.

I saw someone left a couple of donuts, the leftovers from a dozen. I noticed there were some metal scraps next to them, and some of the metal had fallen on the donuts. Since I was so hungry, I dusted off one of the contaminated donuts and ate it anyway.

A few hours after I ate the donut, I found myself in a lot of pain. I went to lie down in an empty student lounge. During the prior three years, I had never become sick.

I continued to suffer for a month. In February 2006, the acute pain in my abdomen was mostly gone, though not entirely. After the pain would subside in late February, it would return again with a vengeance, and be sustained and intense. Besides the pain in my abdomen, I did not have other symptoms. Even today, the pain is not completely gone.

§

I began hearing voices on the last weekend of January 2006, though I told no one. I believe it was a Saturday, about one month after eating the contaminated donut. I do not know whether it was related to eating the metal scraps or if it would have happened anyway.

That January, about one year ago, I heard voices as vividly as any live person talking to me, though they were inside my mind, and I was awake. The first time I heard voices, I heard a group of university students making fun of me for my homelessness from a long distance. Initially, I thought their voices were real.

During the following two months, I would no longer be able to hide in the university area.

CHAPTER TWENTY

As I sit here in the rose garden this day, in January of 2007, I reflect on how I have been homeless now for nearly four years.

I have suffered severe abdominal pain from accidently ingesting the metal scraps a year ago. But otherwise, apart from a couple of mild colds, I have still never been sick. During this last year, from February 2006 until now, I have slept outside almost every night. I often feel resilient and healthy while sleeping outside.

I still feel like life is a video game, and I am trapped in it. Because I have no permanent place to live, no job or formal studies, I feel like I have escaped from the video game. My mind is too cloudy, every day, for me to work, even if I wanted to. But I cling to my decision to remain independent from family and friends, and to not seek their help. I vow to never work a job or go back to school. I know working or attending classes would make me feel as though I were trapped in a hellish reality.

Because no one seems to say anything about how I search for leftover food, I have begun doing it much more often. Searching for food is sometimes discouraging and horrible. But since I have become shameless about looking for it, I sometimes enjoy finding things.

From March 2003 until now, while I have been homeless, I have experienced constant exhilaration and optimism. For years, I have eaten leftover salads from the big university lunch cafeteria, small unfinished sandwiches, and people's abandoned half-drunk sodas. I find gourmet coffee. If I have trouble finding food, I drink an excess of soda pop, which is everywhere. It keeps me going until I can find a time and place to search for more food.

Sometimes, I wonder if the abdominal pain I still suffer is a hallucination or completely real. I believe it is real. It has lessened slowly over the last few months, but I still feel pain. Having a full stomach helps alleviate the pain.

§

While living as a homeless person, I used to watch the sunrise. Experiences like these have made up for the normal life I am missing.

The window from the second floor of a university science building enabled me to see the prettiest and most vivid pink clouds. I would open the window blinds and watch for several minutes. Climbing to the top of a parking garage allowed for a great view of the turquoise mountains at dawn. I never considered that the parking garage where I watched the sunrise was private property, and that I should not have been there. Today, I no longer climb to the top of the parking garage in the mornings because I am worried that I might be arrested.

§

I no longer resemble the student I once was. I have become like a catatonic animal. I know I spend way too much time watching sunrises, sunsets and the night skies. Every day, I feel strong, deep emotions. I am always alone when I watch nature, and I love being alone during these times when I am thinking and daydreaming for hours. As time passes, I have become more and more alone. I have gone for days and weeks without seeing anybody I know.

It is as though I am unaware I am really homeless, and living on food I scavenge. Somehow, my clouded mind is producing feelings of exhilaration to comfort me, and it feels wonderful.

§

Despite my homelessness, March 2003 up until now has been a period of my life characterized by much study, fundraising for Africa, travel, and meeting new friends. It was Saturday, January 28th, 2006, when everything changed. That day, I began hearing a large crowd of students yelling out about how I was a "homeless hoodlum." I could not tell where the voices were coming from, and I kept looking around for a small crowd of people. The hallucination was new to me. I could not immediately tell whether the voices I heard in the distance were in my mind or real. But somehow, I did not care.

If it had happened in real life, I would have felt bullied. But when I heard the hallucination of students that day, I somehow liked having all the attention, even though their comments were derogatory.

A few days later, I was taking a shower at the apartment of some of my few university friends when I heard a group of men making fun of me. They were talking about me loudly and saying over and over again that I was a "homeless hoodlum" and that I was naked.

I thought the men were looking at me through an open window in the bathroom, but I looked over and over the bathroom and found no window. There was only a wall where the noise was coming from. I thought that if others had come into the bathroom, they would also have been able to hear the men. But afterward, when I was certain there was no window or sunroof, I slowly realized it had been a hallucination.

At the same time that I began experiencing this altered reality, I began to hear voices inside of my mind. They were different than my other hallucinations. The voices were as real as a dream. I did not physically hear them, but knew what they were saying. The voices were like laugh tracks in a sitcom which the audience hears but the actors do not. In the same way, the voices were in a different dimension than my reality. Like actors cannot hear laugh tracks, I knew other people could not hear the voices.

The voices were also similar to the experience of having a recurring thought in one's mind. When they appeared in January 2006, they first began to repeat my thoughts to me. If I thought "tomorrow I hope to" they would invade my thoughts, repeating to me the phrase "tomorrow I hope to," like an echo. They soon became independent and said many things, and anything. The voices came on slowly, and they took about two months to really affect my life. After about two months, in March 2006, I began hearing them all the time.

§

Like the first hallucination I experienced in the shower, I continued to hear other people's voices. They never spoke to me, but about me. It was like being on a bus with a rude person in the back who is speaking about another person shamelessly and loudly. I sometimes thought that other people could also hear when I had these hallucinations. Fortunately, the hallucinations I experienced in my reality were less frequent and less disturbing than the voices that raged in my mind.

When I began hearing voices, I knew in my heart that something was very wrong, but I was afraid to mention it to other people. I convinced myself that everyone heard voices, and that since no one else was talking about them, I should not either.

I still believe that no matter what happens while I am

homeless, I will eventually be changed back, and no longer feel the cloudiness and fog in my mind. I cling to my belief that the voices will go away on their own after I become successful, and after my time in American poverty ends. The voices even told me that they would eventually go away after I become rich and famous.

Last year, I began to consider traveling again to Europe. I remember how much clearer I was able to think while in Taiwan. All I want is to have the state of mind I had before I heard the voices. Someday, when I successfully arrive in Europe again, I expect the voices will disappear, and I will be healed completely. I often think about going to Europe again, about clothes I will pack to wear there. My other trips in 2004 came about, though they looked impossible. Perhaps going to Europe again will be as easy as my previous two trips to England were.

§

Sometimes it is as though the voices better understand my situation than I do. They occasionally mock me to try to convince me to ask someone for help. The voices began to call me a "hoodlum" all the time, and they shouted to me "Hoodluming! Hoodluming!" over and over again. They said, "Bethany Yeiser is a homeless hoodlum!" at least a hundred times a day, sometimes they still do. It is unbearable.

I sense that the voices are saying this to force me to find a safer place to spend my nights. As they mock me, they continue to mandate I change my living situation. They tell me that if I continue staying outside late at night, I will be assaulted.

Soon after I began to hear the voices, they told me to talk to Scott, my friend who occasionally took me out to lunch. The voices suggested I confess to Scott that something was very wrong, tell him that I have no place to live, and ask him for help. If I did call Scott and confess to him that I am homeless, I am certain he would show up immediately to make sure I have a safe place to stay at night.

Today, I could contact the Chinese family I stayed with in New Mexico, other friends, or my parents. I know my parents moved, and I do not know where they live, but I could find out if I tried. Any of these people would help me immediately. The voices say I badly need to see a psychologist or other medical professional. But though they might sometimes be right, the voices are not intelligent. They are repetitive like a broken record, and they often change and say the opposite thing.

§

In late March 2006, the voices became louder. They began to shout at me whenever I tried to open a book or read anything. When I tried to read, they repeated the words on the page back to me. It was like when they had repeated my thoughts back to me initially.

Once, I was in a library trying to read a book, despite the voices, and I saw several words on the page were underlined once, twice or three times. I turned the page and saw these strange patterns again. Finally, I chose a different book. But even with the next book, I experienced the same bizarre visualization. The lines were as real as any image I had ever seen. When I chose a third book and saw the same lines, I knew I was hallucinating.

I was in a library when I heard a woman with high heels that made a loud noise walking back and forth nearby where I was trying to study. At first, I thought everyone could hear it. But then, I noticed it was too regular and too loud. She walked back and forth without a pause more times than anyone ever would. It was certainly a hallucination.

I have seen other bizarre things. One day I was trying to study in a library again, though unsuccessfully, when a librarian came to ask me a question. When I looked up at him, I saw his face was distorted, twisted and ugly. Because it was so distorted, I knew it was a hallucination, and it was frightening. In late spring 2006, I looked at myself in a mirror one day and saw a picture of the little girl from the Simpsons TV show, Lisa, but with my facial features.

When I occasionally meet old friends on the street in passing, I become frightened, as they often appear to have distorted faces. I try hard to ignore them, hoping they do not see me. On one occasion, I met a friend with a distorted face while walking the campus, and she greeted me. I was able to recognize that it was her, but during our whole conversation, which lasted a few minutes, her face looked ugly and distorted. Another day, I drank a plain coffee that tasted minty, though it was not flavored. I am having audio, visual and even taste hallucinations.

§

I eventually began to hear not just singular voices, but a choir of children's voices in my mind. They observe me and comment on my behavior and life choices, particularly my homelessness. They follow me all the time. Sometimes I hear one little boy's voice or little girl's voice coming out of the choir and above it. With time, I began hearing the voice of a kind grandfather who soon turned into an evil grandfather who wanted me to suffer. There are other characters in my mind, including a grandmother, a politician, and a friendly police officer. Eventually, I began hearing the "savior."

After the little boy and the little girl appeared in my mind, the voices were sometimes complimentary, though ridiculous. They still sometimes reflect that I am fluent in Chinese, which I am not. They say I had a perfect score on my high school SAT test, which I did not. They say I am one of the smartest people in the world, and that along with a few other people, I will have a position of power, which is ridiculous. But when the voices speak to me about how I will later become a great person of success and importance, though it may be ridiculous, it is thrilling. Sometimes they assure me that my dreams of raising money for Africa will come true.

The voices soon began telling me they were "beeping" me. It was like they were a heart monitor. They seemed to be communicating to me that they were as much a part of me as my beating heart. Today, sometimes they just say "beep" over and over again. Then, they suggest that if I just hit myself or scream, I will find relief from hearing them "beep" me. They somehow make me hit myself hard and scream loudly and often, against my will. They take over me, forcing me to behave as I never would.

Even today, I sometimes yell out loudly and without reason because of the voices. Hearing the voices say "beep" again and again as they force me to hit my forehead has been one of the worst experiences of my life. With time, they have become stronger. I sometimes cannot choose to ignore or go against the voices. Sometimes, I feel terrified by what goes on in my mind.

When the voices expanded in character, I began living in an

alternate reality where I could no longer tell what was real. Though I tried to read, the voices would still repeat every sentence back to me. By March 2006, I had become functionally illiterate.

Later on in spring 2006, I tried to meet with some of the few friends I still had who were students. When the voices began in January 2006, they would go away when I met with people.

But the voices began to talk to me or about me, even when I was with others. The voices began taking over my life. I have stopped meeting with the rest of my few friends almost entirely.

CHAPTER TWENTY-ONE

The voices began yelling at me incessantly about how I did not have a place to sleep. I had a few friends who occasionally welcomed me to stay with them for a few days at a time beginning in March 2003 when I lost my home. Today, I occasionally see some of these people. But when the voices appeared in January 2006 they began bothering me without end to stop asking for favors from anyone.

Unable to think, and wanting to escape the voices, I considered sleeping in the churchyard where I live today. I knew homeless people were not asked to leave. I decided to try sleeping by a side door of the church for just one night. Before sleeping at the church, I had not noticed it was beside a dormitory where I lived in 2000 as a student, scoring good grades.

My first night at the church, I met the gardener. He was a kind, middle-aged man. He asked me my name, and I answered him honestly. I cannot remember the details I gave, but I believe I told him I used to be a student at the big university. He asked no other questions and left me alone. Sometimes, I still see him briefly in the mornings. One evening, he gave me a piece of chocolate cake. Even though it has been nearly a full year since I have lived there, he has always left me alone.

§

My first night sleeping at the churchyard, I sat down on a concrete side entrance to the church. I put on two skirts in layers underneath my green dress to stay warm. I found it was quiet. After about half an hour, I saw an opossum walking around about fifty feet away. I saw several cockroaches, but they never bothered me. Since I had experienced hiding in locked buildings and leaving early in the mornings before the janitors arrived, it was wonderful to sleep until six or seven without worry. I enjoyed the fresh air. It was better than the many nights I had spent alone in public bathrooms.

After I stayed outside the church for several days, I found blankets in the bushes near when I slept. Though I did not know it, the blankets must have been left for me or for other homeless people.

Today, after close to a year, I still find the same bedding and sleep in it every night. The blankets were left in a thick plastic garbage bag. When I wake up at six or seven, I fold the bedding, and I store it in the thick garbage bag in case it rains. After I hide the bag in the big green bushes beside the church building, I leave for the day, usually to go to the rose garden.

I still have never viewed myself as like other homeless people who collect garbage and live in homeless shelters or have terrible hygiene. Homeless people live in empty lots and are sleeping vagrants, catatonic and staring into the distance. I am not doing these things. I appear to spend hours a day myself staring into space, but it is how I reflect, and rest. I am not truly catatonic. I try extremely hard to not appear to be homeless. I succeed, and I am normal.

I continue to wash up in public bathrooms that others rarely use. I have been doing it during my nearly four years as a "homeless" person. I remember that I have studied languages, raised money, performed as a violinist, and published research as a biochemist. Homeless people are mentally slow and deficient. I cannot truly be homeless.

I feel satisfied with my choice to live outside. It is like camping. I watch the stars at night, gazing at the Big Dipper and Orion. The feeling of waiting for miracles is thrilling. But how many years must I wait for the "savior"?

§

I was sleeping on the church grounds when the rainy season began a few weeks ago. It is hard to live outdoors in the rain, but I survived it last year. It rained during my first spring at the church, stopped for the summer, and recently resumed.

The only place to go to find shelter from the rain is the front entrance of the church, which has a high, short overhang. To the right of the front entrance is a beehive, though they are only small sweat bees and do not cause very painful stings. When it first rained, I moved to the front of the church with the overhang rather than getting soaked on the side entrance.

Occasionally, there is an older man who sits on the left side of the church entrance in the rain, furthest from the beehive, smoking something. Since I want to stay as far from him as I can but still under the overhang, I sometimes sleep near the beehive. I have been stung three times, but the stings were not severe or painful, just itchy. The older man never spoke to me, came near me, or bothered me, but I am certain he is real. I see him resting at night in one place for hours at a time.

During my ten months living and sleeping outside at the church, I have rarely encountered other people, except for the old man. There was one night when a man came towards me and lay down beside me. I screamed as loud as I could. He hesitated but left after about a minute. Another night, very late when I was trying to sleep, a man came and lay down on top of my blankets, on top of me. I did not know what to do, so I decided to play dead. He left quickly. Up until today, no one else has bothered me.

As my days at the church have become months, I continue to suffer from auditory and visual hallucinations. These hallucinations give me experiences as real as anything I have ever seen, heard, or experienced. I become overwhelmed with bad, gross smells. With time, the hallucinations have become more frequent and irritating, and I continue to hear the chorus of children's voices every day.

Sometimes I see people who make faces at me to try to get my attention as I walk around on the streets. Other people I see who have strange faces look away and never acknowledge me. Others are friendly. I very rarely speak to any of the people I see with distorted faces.

I was near the university campus one day when I saw a Chinese friend standing at an intersection near an apartment building, waving at me. At first, I thought everyone could see her. But seconds later, I noticed she was behaving like a waving character in an amusement park. I realized that she was not real. Not only had she returned to China months prior, but she would never have stood at an intersection continually waving like a machine.

I have seen visual hallucinations of people from other times of my life, such as a former research advisor and an old violin teacher.

§

As time passes, I have begun to see normal animals, such as

birds, begin to look like mechanical animals. I remember watching one of the "mechanical birds" one morning on the campus. Sometimes, I consider whether the whole earth is actually like Disney World, full of mechanical animals and buildings which are actually just created pictures in the distance. I sometimes wonder if there are secretive people who control various mechanical illusions for the community to see, while never disclosing their work to any person. Sometimes, I am preoccupied with the question of whether the church I sleep next to is actually just four walls with emptiness inside.

I wonder why the people who control these illusions and machines never speak of their work and do everything in secret. I wonder whether I am mentally slower than everyone else, as I guess everyone else knows of these truths by the time they are in high school or college. I reason that everyone in society who is old enough to have this knowledge must never speak of these truths, or as punishment, they will be deemed insane.

Something inside of me is determined to keep these new revelations a secret, and I keep my new understanding of the world as much of a secret as if I did not know these new things. It is what everyone else seems to be doing. But sometimes, something deep inside of me is skeptical, and wonders if the new findings about how the world works are untrue.

§

I met Anne, a young Caucasian woman, in late spring 2006. She was the wife of a student at the university, and a friend of some of my acquaintances. Despite having lost nearly all of my friends, I saw that Anne was a kind and intelligent girl, and I wanted badly to have her friendship.

Soon after I met Anne, I told her I was doing "independent study," and I mentioned some of my language studies and needs in passing. Though I could no longer study at all, I told her I was studying the foreign languages. I wanted it to still be true.

Over the years, I never revealed how desperate I was to anyone, even Anne. Though Anne barely knew me, she was compassionate. She took me grocery shopping and paid for everything, and she gave me a few hundred dollars to buy food.

It was hard to buy food without a refrigerator or place to store it. It seemed Anne had no idea what my situation really was, though she had certainly heard rumors that I wanted a permanent place to stay. I began going to the grocery store daily to buy food with the money Anne deposited in my bank account. It was cheaper than the local cafeteria.

Soon after I met Anne, she invited me to a party. I tried as hard as I could to ignore the voices long enough to make myself presentable to attend. While at the party, I thought I looked decent, but I was aware that my hair was still oily. Whenever I washed it, I was still using hand soap. A few months into 2006, my hygiene had worsened. I needed help to find a normal place where I could take a shower. I hoped Anne was blind to my poor hygiene.

While I was with Anne's friends, another young woman took out a laptop computer and said she was using a "wireless" connection to go online. I had never seen a "wireless" connection like that before, and I do not know how she was able to connect to the Internet, if she were even on the Internet. I still wonder if she was pretending to go online in an effort to make fun of me.

One day, I received an email from Anne inviting me and a few other girls who were mutual friends to spend the night in her apartment. I went, and at first, I was having a wonderful time. But when Anne showed me her wedding pictures, I saw people I had stayed with in Kenya. This included many pictures that were of my Kenyan host, Naomi, who I lived with in Nairobi for a few weeks. I wondered if her wedding photos were manipulated to communicate something to me about my experience in Africa, but I did not know what it all meant. I decided to ignore it, and to not say a thing to my friends about it.

During times when I am sure I am hallucinating, it seems no one else can tell. Even today, no one has ever asked me if I am hallucinating. Today, I believe that when I saw Anne's wedding pictures, I was hallucinating.

§

One evening, Anne invited me to join her and a couple of her friends at a sushi restaurant in the downtown area. She picked me up and paid for everything. That night, after dinner, I asked her to drop me off by an apartment complex where I was telling friends I lived. I planned to stay there for about half an hour before leaving for the churchyard to sleep there, as I always did. The apartment complex was only a five-minute walk from the church.

But that night, after Anne dropped me off, there were people in the complex who did not know me. I felt pressure to quickly leave the complex where I had hoped to hide. I cannot remember the details, but after I left the apartment where I did not live and headed for the churchyard, I believe Anne followed me down the street in her car.

Minutes after I arrived at the church, I saw a car similar to Anne's pull up. A person from the car walked a few steps into the churchyard, looked in my direction, and then looked around her to the right and to the left. Then, she held up her hands as though she did not know what to do. It was as though the person were confused and upset. I honestly do not know whether the person I saw that night in the distance was a hallucination, or really Anne. But I do believe Anne found out that night that I was living in the churchyard.

After seeing Anne on the church grounds, I simply ignored her. I pulled the garbage bag stuffed with my bedding out of the bushes and lay down to sleep on the bedding, as always, on the concrete entrance beside the church. But when I tried to sleep, I heard a group of women loudly talking on the other side of the side entrance door. I had never heard the women there before, though I had slept on the side entrance for months. I was surprised they had noticed me. The women seemed annoyed by my presence by the door, and they thought my presence there was inappropriate. But they also seemed excited about me. As they talked about me, they alluded to my bright future, though they were sometimes referring to me as a "hoodlum."

I kept looking at the door beside me. But there was no window, and the group of women behind the door could not be seen. I was certain the voices of the women would have been audible to anyone who was lying where I was.

I heard the voices of the women talking about me that night until the early hours of the morning. When I heard them, they somehow eliminated the embarrassment and pain I felt when Anne found out I was homeless.

The voices in my mind had always told me before to seek help and change my situation, but that night, they assured me that living as a homeless person was the right thing. They sounded interested in my bright future, and were louder than usual. I learned from the voices that the women sleeping behind the door to the side entrance had been there every night, though I did not know this before. I had never heard them before.

For the first time, I heard my brother in my mind. I discovered that he had been a student at the university, though I had not known this before. My brother excitedly told me that he had been waiting for me to emerge as a national celebrity, and that he was helping to create and direct the voices.

I heard the "savior" for one of the very first times. I had been hoping and waiting to hear from him for so long. He assured me he was coming to meet me soon. I was surprised at how young he sounded, roughly my age. I thought he would be older.

Before I fell asleep, at perhaps three A.M., I saw that newspaper reporters who heard about my upcoming fame arrived at the churchyard. I noticed a bright flash when they took a photograph of me as I lay there. I was expecting to see it in the newspaper the next day.

§

I woke up the next morning thrilled that the women inside the church entrance thought I had a bright future, and happy that I had met so many new people in my mind. Sometimes, today, I am still amazed at the way humans are able to connect and speak to each other through their thoughts. That morning, with some reluctance and nervousness, I looked in both school and city newspapers, but found no photograph or article. I eventually realized that the photographer's flash was a hallucination.

I never thought about whether the women and the new people I met in my mind were hallucinations or real. The hallucinations were becoming the best and worst parts of my life. Even today, when I experience a crowd of voices predicting my success, I forget that at other times, they say the opposite, and are derogatory.

I was exhausted from staying up late, since the night's hallucinations kept me awake. I went to the rose garden, hoping no one would notice me resting or sleeping in one of the gazebos. The voice of the friendly police officer character in my mind assured me that it was okay just for one day.

§

The idea that I might be mentally ill has entered my mind. But I know I am different than schizophrenics I have heard about. Schizophrenics are weak people who cannot handle their problems and whose behavior is bizarre. My experiences do not match the stories I have heard about schizophrenics. To this day, the voices feel like a personal problem. I think of how I scored great grades before, and successfully studied Hebrew and Chinese, unlike any homeless or schizophrenic person I know of. Mentally ill people have poor cognition.

Although I was having problems, I was smart, and I imagined Anne might try to bring my friends together to confront me about my homeless situation. I was careful to never see all of my friends at the same time to prevent it. I reasoned if one of my friends somehow contacted my family, I could break my relationship off with that person only and keep the rest of my friends.

About the time Anne probably found out I was homeless, she offered to pay for a flight for me to return to Ohio. She seemed to have no idea that I was homeless. Though she offered, I was not interested. I knew I could not go back to the Midwest. I was still waiting for a miracle to happen so I would have lots of money and be nationally famous, and so that my mind would clear. I thought now and then about my next trip to Europe. Today, I hope I will be going to France.

I saw Anne once or twice after the sushi dinner. Soon after, the voices were bothering me so much that I was too distracted to meet with almost anyone. I lost touch with Anne.

CHAPTER TWENTY-TWO

With every passing month, the voices have become louder and more intolerable. I have begun hearing new characters such as a politically powerful middle-aged woman. The "savior" talks to me more frequently. He assures me everything I am doing is right. To this day, I find it amazing that I can converse with him in my mind, though we have not met in reality.

My auditory, visual and olfactory hallucinations are getting worse, but I know I am still a normal person in my appearance and actions. I am not behaving like a homeless person. I cannot really be homeless.

I have never stopped trying to read at the libraries. Unlike the schizophrenics I have heard of, I have always loved to read heavily and about all kinds of things, including current events overseas. But I am still unable to concentrate.

During summer 2006, I browsed the Internet, but saw things online that made no sense. One day, I was reading an online newspaper article about a Chinese celebrity, and the newspaper listed the Chinese name of one of my friends as the celebrity, in Chinese characters. Knowing that the name in the newspaper was a hallucination and that I was "seeing things," I felt afraid.

Early one morning, on my way to a library, I looked at the name of the library building and saw that the letters on the brick wall had changed. The name of the library on the front of the brick building was one letter different, with the "B" of the first word changed to a "C."

§

When the voices started in January, a year ago, they were mostly talk, making commentary on my actions. Initially, they filled my mind, and I was unable to concentrate. With time, the voices became less talk and more commands. By summer 2006, they began controlling my behavior. As I walked the university area, they began telling me which streets to turn on and different places to go. They demanded I search for food whenever I was hungry, even if other people were near and might see. They mandated I take walks in inappropriate places like along big roads where there were almost never pedestrians. They demanded I spend more time in libraries, though I cannot read.

Today, sometimes they make irritating noises that cause me to scream or yell out in public while I walk the neighborhood. They keep repeating swear words. They tell me there will be relief if I just yell out the same profanity. I never swore before in my life, but because of the voices, I have lost control of myself. The voices are winning, and I start swearing loudly sometimes while walking the streets. As the months pass, going against the voices is becoming impossible.

§

In fall 2006 (I cannot remember the exact date), the voices told me to throw away my dirty old shoulder bag. I carried beautiful light dresses and some of my favorite books. Not wanting to, but driven by the voices, I threw away everything I was carrying, including my state identification and bank card. After I trashed the few belongings I had loved, I possessed nothing. I had only the green dress, and nothing else.

Months prior to throwing away everything, I opened a lock box at the bank. I put all of my paperwork, my passport, and CDs with electronic copies of documents in the box. I left enough money at the bank to pay for the box before I threw away both my bank card and the key.

§

I cannot always counter the voices. Ideas that I would normally consider to be ridiculous or even wrong become acceptable when the voices say they are acceptable. The voices still lead me to scream in public, walk in places where I am not supposed to be, and behave in other ways that are bizarre. In October 2006, the voices led me to walk to the downtown area and then walk back and forth between intersections. Though I did not mean to attract attention to myself, some people noticed that I looked lost and confused, and possibly disruptive. Others probably noticed my unusual green dress.

I was arrested by police and taken to jail twice, in October 2006 and again the next month over Thanksgiving Day. Both times when I was arrested, the voices were raging in my mind.

The first time I was arrested was on October 16, 2006, two days after my twenty-fifth birthday. At that point, I had been sleeping on a concrete slab in the churchyard every night for seven months. Though I had slept surprisingly well outside and even enjoyed it at times, all I wanted for my birthday was a more comfortable place to sleep. That day, the voices demanded I try to sleep in a more comfortable place. They screamed at me until I went to a lounge I knew of on the university campus where no one should or would ever sleep. It was a nice lounge area in front of offices. I knew that staying in a university lounge was inappropriate and even wrong, but the voices told me to do it again and again.

The voices said that no one would notice if I were to go rest in the lounge area. They said it was my right as a former student. The voices also tried subtle tactics, offering me the opportunity to stay there as their gift to me for my twenty-fifth birthday. The difficult thing was not the voices' explanations as much as their incessant taunting me. They told me again and again without fail to go there until I was driven by them to do it. It was night when I arrived there, and everyone was gone. That night, no one noticed. I slept in the lounge and left early in the morning of October 14th, my twenty-fifth birthday, which was a Saturday. The voices appeared to have been right.

On Monday the 16th, I went to another lounge area I was familiar with, and where I had often rested without being noticed. I was exhausted. I wanted to go to a friend's house, or even to a nearby park to rest, but the voices told me over and over to avoid my friends. The voices told me to go lay down in the comfortable lounge where I had secretly slept.

The lounge where the voices told me to lay down was primarily for linguistics students. They told me that I was a linguist by some definitions. I was reminded of how studying ancient languages had once been my hobby, and of how I had studied vocabulary and phrases in Chinese. The voices continued their explanations, saying I needed my rest, and they continually taunted me without any relief. They screamed at me and would not stop. I could not escape them, and I could not take it anymore.

I knew it was inappropriate to go to the lounge and lay down there in the middle of the day. Students would be there studying in the lounge, and staff would be working at the adjacent office. But the voices were controlling me. Finally, I was won over by the voices. They just said it too many times. I gave up. I never would have gone there during the day had it not been for voices. My mind had changed, and I followed them.

After a few minutes, I reached the lounge. At the command of the voices, I pulled a cushion off a chair in the lounge and lay on the floor. Within minutes, the city police arrived.

I have little recollection of what happened next. A police officer approached me and was asking me something, I do not remember what, but I could not speak. The voices told me that I was lying too far to the left, and that was why the police were there. They said I needed to listen to their instructions better next time.

A police officer handcuffed me, and he sat me down facing a bright light coming from an athletic facility nearby. I tilted my head around to try to avoid looking at the light. I had never seen a city police car on the campus, even during all my years as a student.

I was taken into a police car with two officers. They seemed rather kind. They were driving me somewhere on an interstate near the university area. Since I was rarely driven anywhere during my homelessness, it was actually fun for me. The voices of the two officers seemed to quiet my fears and make me less intimidated. Like I was a child, I felt I was in good hands. I asked the officers if they would take me back home when the ordeal was over, as I considered my home to be in the university area. They told me yes, of course. I did not realize they were being sarcastic.

There was a night one year prior when I was walking the campus area late at night, and a police officer I saw on the street had kindly offered me rides home. I always trusted the police. On the day of my arrest, as they drove me away from the university in handcuffs, I told them the police had given me rides late at night. I did not realize that telling them about my previous encounters with police was not going to help my case. I did not understand what was happening to me.

§

When the police officers arrived at a place about a fifteen-minute drive away, they took off my handcuffs and put me in a small cell (about fifteen feet by fifteen feet) that had a glass window looking out on the hall. Several police officers went by, and I thought they were making faces at me. The faces of the officers were not distorted like my hallucinations. Because of the fear I felt, my hallucinations disappeared, and I am sure their condescending faces were real.

It seemed the officers thought they had finally captured me and were victorious. I had a feeling in my heart that I had done nothing wrong, so their faces did not bother me at all. I knew I could not contradict the will of the voices. Even when I tried with everything I had, I could not go against them. I felt that any feeling of victory on their part must have been a mistake because I was doing nothing wrong. I believed that God had ordained for me to be in jail at that time, and that it was somehow part of his plan for my life.

There was no toilet in the cell, and fortunately, I did not need to use it. I would not have used it anyway in a place where men were looking in so often.

After several minutes, a police officer handed me a clipboard with papers and asked me to describe the events leading up to my arrest. The officer had been with me in the police car, but it was not until I was put in the cell that I saw his face for the first time. He was an older man with bright blue eyes, and he seemed kind, which I found comforting. I felt relieved.

After the officer gave me the clipboard, he told me, sarcastically, to write about how I trusted the police, how they had given me rides home before, and how I had a great relationship with the local police. I still felt he was in it for my best interest, but somehow, writing about my former experience knowing and trusting local police officers seemed to be inappropriate when I was asked about the events leading up to my arrest.

The fear I felt while being picked up by the police continued to weaken my hallucinations. I managed to write a few paragraphs about my time as a student at the university years ago, and how I believed that I was still welcome there.

Half an hour after I was placed in the small cell, two officers took me to a female corrections facility, though I cannot remember traveling there. Upon my arrival, the officers asked me if I needed to go to the medical clinic for any reason or needed any medications. They informed me that I would not have another opportunity to get medical help.

I was shocked by how many women I saw in the medical clinic area. I wondered what medications the women needed and why. I saw at least one woman getting a shot, and I was amazed that she would actually ask for it. I wondered what was wrong with her. If she needed to see a doctor, why was she in jail?

A few minutes later, I was put in a cell about ten feet by fifteen feet, in a hallway with perhaps three other similar cells. It had a small bench where two or three women were sitting, a toilet, and a small drinking fountain. There was no room to sit anywhere, except to squeeze in behind the toilet. Fortunately, it was clean.

I remembered a time when I was on my humanitarian trip to Nairobi, and the local papers reviewed the case of an innocent man who was picked up by police. He was made to spend the night beside a filthy toilet in a jail cell, so similar to me. I remembered what I learned in high school and during all of my education growing up about arrested people getting trials right away. I thought I would be given a toothbrush, a shower, and a short time outside every day. But none of these things happened. I thought I would be in a much larger space, but I was packed into a tiny cell. I was shocked that I was put into a tiny cell with three other women.

Months had elapsed since I began sleeping secretively on grounds of apartment complexes in the early morning hours. No one had ever noticed me at night. After that, I spent every night for seven months on a concrete slab of the side entry of a church. That night in jail, I squeezed behind the toilet and put my head down on the ceramic cold floor at the base of the toilet, and I fell into a deep sleep after only a few seconds. I slept better than I imagine most people do in nice hotels. There was just this rare feeling that here in the cell, I was safe.

I woke up once or twice when the other women used the toilet, which made me move. Afterward, I immediately fell asleep in the same place, each time within seconds. One woman asked a female officer for a tampon, and the officer came back with one. I listened to one woman speak to another woman while I was briefly awake, and I discovered that one of them was incarcerated on a DUI charge.

Later on, the noise of a cart rolling down the hallway awakened us. I wondered what was happening, but it sounded like food was being served. I do not remember how I knew this, but it was about four o'clock in the morning. To my disbelief, I was given a restaurant-style breakfast of a delicious hot egg omelet and sausage. I took a bite of the breakfast, and I could not remember the last time I had eaten a warm, prepared breakfast. Though I often found good leftover food, it was always cold. It had been a few months since I had a hot breakfast, and in pure gratitude to God who I believed had taken me to the jail at that time for a purpose, I almost began to cry. I realized there were some definite benefits to being in jail over being on the street.

From my arrest onward, the voices had been more or less silent. It was as if they were distracted. I wish that the police officers could have seen what was happening in my mind and identified me as a confused person rather than a criminal.

§

A police officer led me out of the crowded cell for a brief time and made me give ink prints of my fingers and thumbs on top of a large machine. In my confusion, I began to believe that the ink used in the fingerprinting would later give me a terrible disease, which I thought was the real reason they were taking my fingerprints. I thought that, like the big machine, my body was also a machine, and now the two of us shared the same fingerprints.

A female officer made me stand for a picture in front of two bright lights. I wondered if the light would later cause me to have eye problems, and I wondered if that were the real reason they were using the bright lights.

An hour after breakfast, an officer led me down to a lower level where she gave me mattress pads to sleep on. The darkness there was a true nightmare. It was like a movie where prisoners are taken to dark dungeons, without even a ray of light. There was no natural light. I could not sleep, since I had already slept so well in the cell. About thirty people were down there.

The darkness in the cells continued to be a nightmare without any relief. Officers moved us from here to there, different rooms every few hours during what I believed to be about a day. All were dark.

Some were crowded like I would not have believed if an American had told me, like the first cell I shared. It was as though each woman had five square feet or less of space, and there were often about thirty women. I cannot remember the food given at other times. I do remember that I received the exact same breakfast the next morning as I did the first day. It was less fulfilling when the same food was given a second time.

I was never afraid of darkness before, but the darkness in the jail was overwhelming. One time we were allowed to go into a small room with some real sunlight. There were a few small tables in the room, each with four stools. But the other women frightened me, and I was afraid something would happen if I sat down with them, so I did not enter the room with the natural light during the fifteen minutes we were allowed in. Through the whole time, I kept waiting for that short time that I heard about on TV shows and movies where the prisoners are allowed to go outside, run around and see the sun. I found that it never came, at least not during my time in jail that October. Though I was in the jail at least two nights, I was never given an opportunity to brush my teeth or take a shower.

I cannot remember getting another ride to a different jail building. But after a couple of days, I was transported to a courthouse far away. I later found it to be walking distance from the university area. Before I was released, an officer escorted me into a bright room filled with people where I signed a document stating that I would return for a hearing in early December. I signed it, though I had no idea how I would return. Since the voices had told me to throw away my state ID, I still had no identification. Except for the green dress, I had no clothes.

After I signed the document to return for my court date, I had to wait a long time until the officers let me out of the building. Finally, they returned the shoelaces and earrings they had confiscated from me. I was with another woman who I was surprised to find friendly. After about an hour, they released us out to the center of the city.

The woman I was with greeted a nice man who had come to meet her after she was released. I do not know when or where she made the phone call to plan to connect with him. When we were let out, I did not really know what to do or where to go. She seemed concerned about me. I eventually realized I was in a familiar part of the downtown, and it was about a half hour walk to the area surrounding the university, which I still considered to be my home. Beginning the long walk back home to the churchyard was the only realistic option I could think of.

I could not readily find a place in the center of the city to sit down and tie my shoes, so I just began the long walk without the laces in my shoes. As for my earrings, I feared the police deliberately contaminated them, so I threw them away.

It was evening when I was released. I can hardly remember other times when I was downtown in the evening, and the sunset was truly beautiful. I saw the deep pink dusk, and the turquoise mountains under the radiant pink sky, vibrant in the day's last light. When it became dark, I saw the colored lights of the skyscrapers and the first stars. I felt I was in heaven. I experienced an unadulterated, lovely world. I felt truly set free.

When I reached the churchyard where I had been sleeping almost every night, I felt great relief. I re-laced my black shoes, and I discovered the bedding I hid in the garbage bag behind the bushes days before was still there. I was greatly thankful for my bedding. I lay down on a familiar slab of concrete to go to sleep with my pillow and blanket. Fortunately, it was no longer the rainy season, and there was generally no rain in October. That night, I slept as well as anyone might sleep in a safe campground on a holiday, if not better. I had returned home.

CHAPTER TWENTY-THREE

When I was released from jail, I continued sleeping well outside. I awoke early each morning and walked near the campus and then to the rose garden. The campus was visible in the distance, but I stayed out. I would never walk the campus again because I did not want to risk another incarceration. I enjoyed the beauty of the mornings as I discreetly looked for food left behind by students or other people in the surrounding community.

Soon, the voices led me, once again, to walk to the downtown area of the city. Though I would be alone on busy streets where few people walked, wandering aimlessly, the voices controlled me. I stared with catatonia at beautiful things. The mountains were still crystal clear and blue, and the sky was a lighter blue that stretched far beyond and above the mountains. The strong feelings and the voices drowned out my ability to be reasonable and think about where I was walking. I must have appeared to be lost.

One day in October, while walking, I realized I was in a part of the city that looked rundown, and that I did not know where I was. I had accidently wondered into a dangerous area. Suddenly, while realizing I was in a bad area, I felt a knife or a thick needle stab me in the dead center of my back, and it was extremely painful. I screamed louder than I ever had before. Because it was in the dead center of my back, so accurate, and because no one was near me, I knew the pain was a hallucination. But knowing it was a hallucination made no difference. It was more severe than any pain I had experienced in my life, as horrible as a sting from a wasp.

Going to jail twice after being driven by voices was the worst thing I have experienced during my years as a homeless person, and during my life. But, to this day, the painful hallucinations have been a close second.

The painful hallucinations did not begin until fall 2006, several months after I began hearing voices for the first time. I first experienced the painful hallucinations sometime between my first and second times in jail. During the months that have followed, I have never experienced as much pain as I did the first time I was "stabbed," but today I often feel lesser painful sensations. I usually experience a painful sensation every day or two. Though I am feeling less pain than I had suffered on my first tactile hallucination, the pain I feel is still horrible, and it is slowly growing worse.

My experience of this continuous pain is the only experience over the years that almost led me to ask for medical help. It has become nearly too painful to live with. I have no idea what a doctor or other medical professional might do for me with my hallucinations. I imagine medications for this problem do not exist. But there are police and other officials everywhere, and I could easily ask to be taken to a clinic or hospital. Though I have come close, I have never asked for help.

In addition to experiencing being stabbed in the dead center of my back, I have felt painful sensations in my head, hands, and feet. Whenever I feel the shooting pain, I often scream or loudly yell out. As my painful hallucinations have become a daily ordeal, I constantly hear the choir of children's voices.

§

I no longer know or see almost anyone from my years as a student at the university, from 1999 until 2002. However, one day, I met a young woman in the university area and recognized her as one of my neighbors from my freshman year honor's dormitory in 1999. When we saw each other by chance, she came up to me and asked if I were Bethany from the dormitory. Because I was embarrassed by my appearance and situation, I denied I had ever met her.

One night she came to the side entrance of the church where I was sleeping. I saw her coming, and I buried my face under my blanket and ignored her. But she still walked up to me, and when she came within a few feet of the church entrance, she began speaking to me. She was not concerned about me, but was mocking me.

She recounted her experiences during the day as though she were reading an entry from her diary. As I lay there not acknowledging her, she told me a dirty story that lasted a few minutes. I continued to pretend I was asleep, and I did not move or respond to her at all. She seemed to think seeing me stay at the church was bizarre, and it was as though she almost could not believe it. I am certain she was real and not a hallucination. She was there too long.

After she talked to me about her day, she placed a large rock on my head. I did not know what she was going to do, and I could not believe it was the same girl from my freshman honors dormitory. But then, she left.

She should not have bothered me, but she did leave a five dollar bill. It was some of the only money I have ever gotten for being "homeless," since I have never begged. (There were only two others who sought me out, approached me, and gave me money. One gave me about $10 on Christmas Day of 2006, and the other $20 in 2006 to buy a pair of shoes when she walked by me and saw mine were ruined).

When I found the five dollar bill the next morning, I did not trust her. I felt certain the money was counterfeit, so I ripped it up and threw it away. She had just been so rude. I reasoned she would never behave as she did and then leave me money. In retrospect, I believe the money was probably real and not counterfeit. It appeared to be real.

§

In late November 2006, a month after being jailed, I was experiencing extreme pain in my back again. It was the same type of pain as before, like someone took a sharp, thick needle, dug it into my spine, and slowly pulled the needle downward or upward. In my pain, I did not know what to do, and I was suffering because of it.

I had always tried to never go to the churchyard unless I was "invisible" as I am at night. But one afternoon, since I was in pain, I went to the churchyard anyway. I just wanted somewhere, anywhere, to lie down for a few minutes and get some relief from the back pain. I was hearing voices and having other auditory hallucinations. I was oblivious to my surroundings.

The voices yelled at me whenever I looked at a newspaper. Without access to news, I had become even more detached from reality. Though I did not know what day it was, I remember thinking it was probably Wednesday of the week before Thanksgiving. It was actually the day before Thanksgiving. I was wrong by a full week.

Minutes after I lay down in the churchyard, two police officers called out to me from the road and asked me where I lived. I was still doing everything in my power to avoid telling anyone I was homeless. When friends asked, I simply pointed to a housing complex for female students close to the church and said I lived there, and with my friends, it always sufficed. When the police asked, I said the same thing automatically, pointing to the certain housing complex for female students. But, that day, one of the officers asked me more questions, including a question about one of the women who ran the housing complex. When he discovered I had no knowledge of her, it was obvious to him that I lied about where I lived.

The two officers picked me up and took me to jail again. I did not know that not having a valid address was sufficient reason to be taken to jail. I was not bothering anyone. I wonder if the officers saw me screaming or hitting myself hours prior (because of the voices) and if they had been looking for me. Even now, I am not certain why I was taken to jail that afternoon.

Fortunately, the officers had arrested me at a time when there would have been almost no leftover food to eat because everyone was home for the holidays. While with the officers, I was distracted, and the painful hallucinations temporarily disappeared.

§

My second experience in jail was very different than my first experience. The jail cell had a television that played a Thanksgiving cooking show and other programs throughout most of the day. An officer gave me a Bible to read, and though I was unable to read, I felt comforted to hold the book. The cell had a door near a window that let in some natural light.

During my second time in jail, I had little trouble with painful hallucinations, probably because I was distracted, again, by the fear I felt while incarcerated. When I would later be released, the painful hallucinations would return again with a vengeance.

I was in a cell for a few days over the Thanksgiving holiday. While in jail, I was allowed to take a shower, but I was afraid because I was extremely dirty underneath my green dress. I did not want anyone to see. Before the women showered, I asked an officer if I could be exempt, and she said yes. I did not take a shower during either of my times in jail.

My second time in jail, I was driven far away from the area nearby the university that I called home. After one day, one of the women was released, and the officers told us it was by lottery. Since we were so far from the university and I had no money, I do not know what I would have done if I had been released from the facility at that time. It was too far for me to walk home. I do not know what I would have done for food in a new place without money.

After a few days, I was driven to another jail, a women's facility. I later discovered it was about five miles from the university and its surrounding area. As we drove along in a large bus, I could see the city. I had a hallucination which made the city appear as a huge ant hill with the people running around and through it like ants.

CHAPTER TWENTY-FOUR

I remember the women's facility well. It was a wide open building with lots of room and natural light. Inside, it had many small rooms with hard benches where the women could sit. When I arrived at the facility, an officer gave me carrot sticks, a sandwich and grape drink. I continued to feel relieved that I did not have to find food on my own.

I met some inmates who were nice people. One woman, probably old enough to be my mother, sat beside me. A few minutes later, she laid her head down in my lap and just rested. Unfortunately, some of the other women used the filthiest language I have ever heard. Like my first time in jail, I was afraid of a few of the other inmates. I was worried they might attack me.

The women's facility had more space than the previous jail I had been to, where the rooms were so crowded that no one was able to move. The big rooms were preferable to the former tiny jail cell.

After waiting for an hour at the new facility, I had to remove my clothes and change into a jail uniform. The uniform was light blue. No one seemed to notice how dirty I was. After I changed, officers gave each of the women bedding to carry to their rooms. Officers assigned us to rooms in pairs. The rooms we had for the night had small windows that were about six inches across and a foot high. My first time in jail, there was little sunlight, and the deprivation was one of the worst things I have ever experienced. I was grateful for the natural light.

At the churchyard, I never had a real bed, and I was not accustomed to sleeping in a bed. After my eight months living outside, I preferred sleeping on something disheveled and hard. That night in jail, I did not bother to make my bed. I wanted to feel freer, like I was "at home" by the church again. I took off my jail uniform trousers to sleep since they were way too tight. I did not know how I would remain in them during the next day. Since my shoes were ruined, ripped apart from the left to the right sole, an officer had given me a pair of flip-flops.

After I was assigned to a room, I met my roommate. She told me that she had been apprehended for drug use, and she would never abuse drugs again. She said she would be in jail for about six months. She seemed harmless. I told her I was in on a trespassing charge. I do not believe I told her I was trespassing at a university where I used to be a student, as it no longer seemed to matter.

§

I soon found the county jail was, in some ways, quite a peaceful place. There was the sunlight, nice beds and games such as checkers drawn onto small tables. People seemed laid back. The green dress I had been wearing while homeless still appeared decent, but was dirty on the inside, so it was wonderful that my uniform was clean. Though the other women did not seem to appreciate the food, I saw it as fancy and gourmet.

My first night in the women's facility, I remember thinking I was ready to stay in this new place, where there was food I did not have to scavenge, and where I had clean clothes. I was thankful we were given warm blankets for the night. I did not have to search the church foliage for my blankets in the garbage bag, hoping every night that no one had taken them during the day, and that they were dry.

§

The next morning when I woke up, I had slept well. I had forgotten, again, about how wonderful it was to sleep in a place that was safe. For breakfast, a staff member gave each woman cheerios with milk and a banana. Since I rarely was able to find bananas or milk while searching for food, I was delighted.

Just when I accepted the idea of staying in jail, minutes after breakfast, an officer called me down for release. After I came down the stairs from my small locked room, a few officers said something like "you were 'trespassing' at a university where you used to be a student?" They determined that I did not belong there. Making a joke, an officer casually used one of the worst swearwords in English, freely swearing not at me, but around me. I made a half smile at him and just turned away. I did not belong with the other people at the jail.

I was released from jail without doing any work. As I was leaving, I saw officers assign duties to the women to perform during the day. I do not know whether I would have been able to work in jail or not. My feelings of fear while in jail had weakened my hallucinations for a few days. But I am certain that after a few more days, the voices and painful hallucinations would have returned.

My second experience in jail was good in some ways, since I had been homeless for so long. But at the very end, when I was walking down a hall to be released, a jail staff member opened a large door quickly and almost hit me hard in the face. She could easily have seriously hurt me, and did not apologize. I wondered if other inmates had been hurt by such negligence. I still trusted the authorities and was surprised.

Before I was released from the facility, an officer led me into a room with a huge washer and dryer where a staff member gave me back my green dress. I was delighted to find the jail staff had laundered it. Everyone's clothes had been washed. I felt sorry for inmates whose clothes were supposed to be dry cleaned and were ruined in the jail's washing machine.

As I changed back into the green dress, the voices returned. I had a fit, walking around out of control, back and forth, swinging my arms around and groaning. The voices were controlling me again. An officer looked into the holding cell where I was groaning, and as he zeroed in on me, he showed a twisted smile. He probably thought I was being disruptive because I wanted attention. Since my hallucinations often disappeared in the presence of distractions, before the officer took me back to jail, seeing him enabled me to regain my composure. I am thankful the officer did not decide to keep me in jail right as I was about to be released.

Only minutes after I had encountered the officer and settled down, I was free on the street. I needed to find food. I immediately began searching for any food that may have been left in the garbage outside the jail.

I am certain that even one additional day of jail life would have brought tremendous grief and restlessness to return back to my homeless life. I believe that the voices and pain would have returned if I had spent a few more days in jail.

§

When I was released from jail for the second and last time, I found myself miles from the churchyard I considered my home. Since an officer threw away my ruined black shoes and gave me a new pair of flip-flops, the flip-flops were all I had on my feet. Trying to walk home, I found myself along a busy road with cars whirling by at over forty miles per hour. It had a sidewalk, but as I walked, I saw almost no one else walking, even for miles. The road had one of the prettiest views I have ever seen of the mountains. I envied the working individuals who drove the road back and forth to work every day.

To get home, I walked for miles toward the downtown, coming closer and closer to the buildings in the distance like a lost animal. Since the streets were numbered, when I got to about Fortieth Street, I knew roughly where I was. When I was near Twenty-Eighth Street, I was close to home.

As darkness approached, the city was lit up for the night, and the Christmas decorations in the downtown and on homes were lovely. I stopped for a few minutes to look out at the skyscrapers. I wished that I could live in the neighborhood.

When I returned home to the churchyard, I became nervous to stay there like before, wondering if police would pick me up again. I took my blanket, which was still in the bushes, and tried a different church. The other church had an entrance right on the street, and everyone could see me. I tried sleeping at the church on the street a couple of times, but that church made the churchyard where I had lived for months look comfortable and pleasant in comparison. Though I did not want to go to jail again, I realized that staying in the same churchyard where I had been for the last eight months was the best I could do. Despite being taken to jail for having no place to stay, I still never considered contacting family or friends.

CHAPTER TWENTY-FIVE

The week after Thanksgiving 2006, when I returned from jail, I began to spend more time in the rose garden, thinking, as I am today. Though I badly want to watch the sunrise again, I know the parking garages are technically private property. I do not want to be in various parking garages alone in the early morning where police could pick me up.

Instead, in the early mornings, I always walk for twenty minutes to the rose garden from the churchyard. The rose garden is the same place I stayed and rested after the night Anne found out I was homeless, and after I hallucinated all night.

There is still dew on the ground and on the roses when I get here. A few places in the rose garden have benches, and the park has gazebos. In the mornings, I see white patches of scattered light all over the grass, and I think of how life is beautiful.

Sitting in the garden enables me to escape the voices to some extent. Unfortunately, my painful hallucinations continue to hit me randomly and at odd times, usually in my back, and they are still getting worse. But when I am in the rose garden, my hallucinations often become more tolerable.

Around lunch time, children come into the garden from nearby schools. I stay away from them, but I greatly enjoy seeing them from a distance. It is fun to watch them play and run around. They usually leave lots of food, and I often eat quite well after they are gone.

While in the rose garden, without meaning to, I have drawn some attention to myself. One day I sat on a bench and remained there thinking about my past for over six hours. I was thinking of Ohio and of my years as a student. I remembered my parents' faces, my violin, Christmases when I was a child, and studying hard in my first years of college. I find myself daydreaming like that again today.

Sometimes in the garden, I remember Africa. I am still certain God is in charge of my life and that this period of poverty and homelessness in my life will end. I am certain that I will have money and possessions again, and be wealthy. I believe I will later be grateful for having had my experiences living without money and homeless in America. I look forward to visiting France someday, and I am certain that I will travel again, and that my mind will clear.

One evening, I sat in the rose garden for several hours until dusk, and the dusk reminded me of the human concept of death. I felt provided for and happy to be alive.

§

Last month, as Christmas approached, I began to make some friends in the rose garden. Most were Hispanic. I tried to remember my college Spanish. I spoke a few words and phrases, but overall, I was not successful. I may have appeared ridiculous. I admit, I can barely think in English.

One of the Hispanic people I met in the garden works as a photographer. He is kind, and often invites me to sit with him and his son, who is about my age, and talk while they are waiting for business. I do not know why he is generous to me, but he often gives me food. Though I am wearing the same green dress most days, he and his son never ask any questions. I have also met a few individuals in a local food court who occasionally give me free food.

§

On Christmas Day, 2006, I walked to the rose garden, as usual, to meditate and pass the time. The voices were bothering me as they always do, but were more irritating that morning. They told me to wander around, back and forth, and back and forth on the sidewalk. A young woman who was jogging on the morning of Christmas saw that I was wandering around and confused. She must have thought I was homeless, and she approached me and gave me about ten dollars. I was embarrassed to receive the money, and I am still not sure why she gave it to me, since I do not look a homeless person. I decided to go drop the money off at the nearest church to help needy people. When I walked the ten minutes to the church from the garden, I found myself missing their Christmas Day service by a few minutes.

I was looking for a miracle on Christmas, and I found myself drawn to a large Catholic church. Entering the Catholic church for the first time felt like my Christmas miracle. Though I had never entered it before, I had seen it was beautiful and like a cathedral. I discovered it was even more beautiful inside.

I had not grown up Catholic, but I loved the beauty of the Catholic buildings with their statues, paintings and stained glass. I do not understand why more Protestants and other Christians do not visit these beautiful buildings to meditate.

Late December, 2006, I began going to the Catholic church every day despite my increasingly bad hygiene. Apart from that, I spent most of my days in the garden. I just wanted to pray. Today, I still feel something in my heart asking me why I can be in touch with many people, like the Hispanic photographer, but not my mom and dad. While I have enjoyed the beauty of the church, I have begun to realize that since I have lost touch with my mom and dad, something must be wrong with me.

One day, the Catholic father approached me and asked me if I were homeless. I simply told him no, that I absolutely was not. I must have appeared to be little more than a tramp that day. But after I told him I was not homeless, he treated me with dignity. I see him occasionally.

While in church, and in the rose garden, something in my heart has been changing. Maybe, soon, I will be ready to see my parents again.

CHAPTER TWENTY-SIX

It is January 2012. Many mornings when I wake up, I remember years ago when I was sleeping at the top of a stairwell in a tall building on the cement. I was afraid of all of the people who loved me most. My illness prevented me from making a phone call to my parents, friends or relatives. Any of them would certainly have allowed me to stay in their homes in a warm bed. Some of them would have let me stay with them for months, or indefinitely.

Sometimes I find myself thankful I began hearing voices. I was homeless, but prior to hearing voices, all definitions and rules used in contemporary psychiatry would render me competent on my own. American laws guaranteed my release from any psychiatric ward where I may have been taken.

I was not yet ill enough to be seen as a person in need of psychiatric treatment. I would later recognize that getting psychiatric treatment would become the miracle I was looking for. It would become the greatest miracle of my life.

§

March 2, 2007 was a difficult day for me. Four years prior, on March 3, 2003, I had lost my apartment and began living as a homeless person. When March 2, 2007, arrived, I did not know the exact date, but I could sense that my fourth year "anniversary" of becoming homeless was near. Though I badly wanted to know the date, I could not check it on a newspaper without hallucinating.

When the morning of March 3, 2007 came, I still did not know what day it was. That morning, the voices were especially irritating and relentless. Minutes after I woke up, I experienced an extremely uncomfortable hallucination, which was like a scratching on my back. The hallucination was the most irritating I had experienced yet. It made me scream loudly, almost as a reflex.

As they often did, the voices encouraged me to find relief by hitting myself. I began ramming my forehead with the palm of my hand. Then the voices told me to find relief by swearing loudly. It had been months since I began hearing voices, and I was shouting profanity.

As I got up that morning, I hoped no one had heard me screaming. In an effort to distract the voices, I ran toward the surrounding neighborhood to look for food. But as I ran toward the neighborhood, the voices told me to run the other way, and then the other way again. I began running in a huge zigzag pattern around the churchyard. Like a robot, I could not escape the commands of the voices. Finally, I gave up looking for food. I walked to a small water spigot on the property to wash my face. At that point I think I screamed back at the voices again, but I cannot remember for certain.

Suddenly, someone I had not noticed before approached and grabbed me. A person who lived in the neighborhood called the police, and I saw two women in bathrobes outside speaking with them. I found myself in handcuffs, again. After a few minutes, the police led me into their car, and the police officers told me they were taking me to be observed in a psychiatric ward.

Being with the police distracted me from having hallucinations. I tried to tell the police that today was a special anniversary for me, or "perhaps it was tomorrow." Not knowing the date but thinking it was a special anniversary did not help me look good.

The officers took me to the same holding cell where I was incarcerated before, but I was only there for a few minutes. They seemed concerned about me and gave me a sandwich. They almost certainly knew that I looked around the neighborhood for food.

While I was eating the sandwich, the officers asked for my parents' phone numbers. When I said I did not know the numbers, they went online to research the contact information. I could see them from the cell as they looked up the numbers for my parents. Minutes after my arrival at the police station, they transported me to a psychiatric assessment ward at the university hospital.

§

While in the psychiatric ward, I eventually discovered it was indeed March 3rd, my fourth year "anniversary" of losing my home. I was confused over why I was taken to the ward on a day when I had expected miracles.

When I entered the psychiatric ward, I found it was strikingly small. There was a huge desk for the staff on its right side, and a small window that appeared to overlook an empty swimming pool. A nurse offered me a shower, and having the privacy and warm water was wonderful. Minutes after I took a shower, a doctor met with me.

During my entire four years as a homeless person, part of me remained sane. Whenever I thought of raising millions of dollars for Africa, I kept it to myself. I felt I had no need to tell others about it because I believed they would someday see it when it happened. I realized it was not acceptable in my social circles to be "homeless." I vowed to never appear homeless and stuck to my resolution. I tried to always behave normally so I would not be seen as a homeless person. But I was proud I had never entered a homeless shelter as though it meant I had never been homeless.

My life may have been easier if I had resigned myself to being homeless. I could have accepted food from food banks, slept in a women's shelter, and had my needs met by an organization that helped homeless people. But while living four years as a homeless person, I never accepted that I was homeless.

My mind was creating voices and hallucinations for months before doctors later diagnosed me with a mental illness at the psychiatric hospital. I had delusions and false beliefs for years before I was diagnosed. I was considered schizophrenic only after the voices and hallucinations altered my behavior, and I began screaming and yelling profanity back at the voices in my mind.

CHAPTER TWENTY-SEVEN

That Saturday at the psychiatric assessment ward, I knew it was spring, and that I would be missing the new blooming flowers in the garden. I knew I was missing my older Mexican friend, his son, and the friends they introduced me to who walked the parks and the garden. I told my psychiatrist that I "wanted to go home," but offered no details. I said I had a place to stay. I wanted to convince the psychiatrist that I had no mental issues and was happy with my living situation, which I thought was none of his business. I told him I was fine. I expected that staff would accept my convincing lies that I had a safe place to live, since it was what I always told everyone, and everyone seemed to believe me. But this time they did not.

I did not realize how far I had fallen. My clothes were dirty. I had lost some weight again. My hair was messy. Apart from my Hispanic friends, I had not seen any friends for months. The Mexican people I spent time with had ignored my dirty appearance out of kindness. Looking back, I cannot believe how kind they were to me in my homeless condition. While praying at the Catholic church, I kept to myself, but my Hispanic friends went out of their way to talk to me.

The voices were bothering me while I was being observed in the ward. When I got there, a staff member gave me water from a tap rather than bottled water. I knew the water was not contaminated, but the voices were screaming at me that it was. When I told the staff I wanted bottled water, they told me the tap water was safe and seemed annoyed.

The doctor asked if he could speak with my parents. After having meditated at the church for about two months, I had begun to see the right thing to do was to have my parents in my life again. Since I was being observed in a psychiatric ward, I realized something was wrong with me. Though I would initially refuse medication, I wondered if I needed counseling. That morning, the voices told me to go along with what the doctor asked me to do, which included letting him speak with my parents. The main reason I allowed the doctor to speak with them was because the voices told me to.

A great conflict was taking place in my mind while the psychiatrist and staff observed me. I was still afraid of my parents' involvement in my life, and I wanted to continue waiting for miraculous money to come in for Africa. I still wanted to wait for the "savior," who I fervently believed was coming, and who I still expected would donate millions of dollars and marry me. I had not doubted his coming for over four years. But when I was in the psychiatric ward, the possibility that he might not be coming entered my mind. I never told anyone about him until I wrote this book.

Later on, after I was transferred to a psychiatric hospital, the voices would tell me not to take any medications.

§

For years, I planned on being married, wealthy, and having my own children before I got in touch with my mom and dad again. I imagined I knew the number of girls and boys I would have someday and had thought of names. My illness sometimes gave me other illusions besides expecting my husband and children, including illusions of knowing about the future. After returning from Africa, I clung to the belief that I would become rich and famous.

I was sure that, someday, my parents would admit that I was right to have lost touch with them for a few years. I was certain how I was living was right. I thought I was pleasing God by giving almost all my money away to Africa and other countries, and by taking trips to learn more about the poor. I believed working or going back to school would pull me away from my life of prayer and expectation. I thought I was not truly a homeless person and believed I was very different than any homeless person I had ever seen.

The day I was observed by the psychiatrist, a staff member contacted my mom. He asked me if I wanted to speak to my parents. I felt guilty about speaking to my mom and dad in my current state. I thought of the great love they gave me my whole life, and how badly they wanted to be in touch for my 21st birthday in fall 2002, right after I cut them off. I was twenty-five years old. During all of the four and a half years we were apart, I had ripped up so many of their cards and checks. I thought of how I saw my dad on campus in 2003 and ran away after he saw me and tried to greet me.

But I knew that my parents loved me, and that even after I was taken by police to be observed by a psychiatrist, they would still want me back. Even after not being in touch for four and a half years, I knew my parents would treat me with dignity. I was sure they would overlook the fact that I was in a psychiatric observation ward. That was just the kind of people they were.

Something in my heart was finally ready to hear from my mom and dad. Though I did not want my parents to see me as I was, I decided to give them the opportunity to speak with me if they wanted to. The staff were surprised that I had no idea what my parents' phone numbers and address were, since my parents moved across town after I lost touch with them. The doctor used the information obtained at the police station to call my parents.

After the doctor spoke with my mom, he asked me if I wanted to speak with her. For the first time in four and a half years, we spoke. Her familiar voice was kind and she seemed delighted to hear my voice. Though I was disoriented and desperately ill, she wanted to hear all about how I was. She told me I was her best friend. The point was not that I had been her best friend in the past. She said that I *was* her best friend, and she said she missed me.

I felt her deep love for me. She was not angry, and did not want to get even with me for past wrongs. She seemed so relieved and happy to hear my voice over the phone.

We were not able to talk long because the doctor wanted to see me again.

§

While I was at the psychiatric assessment ward, my parents called the doctor and explained that I had a long history of odd behavior since returning from Africa in 2002. Additionally, staff saw my bizarre reluctance to drink tap water (since the voices told me regular water was contaminated), my fake address, and evidence that I was homeless, which led them to believe I was mentally ill. The staff also saw that though I had not been in touch with my family for a few years, I spoke to them as though it were no problem. They determined I needed psychiatric treatment. At three or four o'clock in the morning of March 4th, EMTs transferred me from the observation ward to a psychiatric hospital. The hospital was run by the university I used to attend.

When I arrived at the psychiatric hospital, a nurse put me in a small, private room with a half-bathroom. It had a window overlooking a small yard with succulent plants and a tall tree. I was greatly disappointed that I was taken to a real psychiatric hospital. But somehow, I found myself at peace, and calm.

Soon after being admitted to the hospital, I was told I had schizophrenia, but I cannot remember who told me or how I was told. Though I was pressured to begin medication, no one sat down with me and explained what my illness was and how it was affecting my life, or at least not that I remember. I was so convinced I was not mentally ill that I would not have listened to them anyway.

Schizophrenia can turn individuals into other people. This is because it involves a change in chemical balances in the brain. For years, I had felt a sadness as though a close friend had died only days prior. The sadness never went away. It was rooted in what I had seen in Africa, but after nearly five years, the acute emotional pain should have weakened. I should have been able to process the difficult things I saw there.

In 2007, I was not the same person as the teenager who played the violin or the girl who attended college in 2001. I was not even the same young woman who visited Africa and Taiwan. But I was certain I did not have schizophrenia or any other mental illness. I thought of the cognition required to create a nonprofit organization and fly all over the world learning about the poor. I thought of the money I had raised for Nairobi. I remembered my past working in the biochemistry lab, and as a violinist, and I considered difficult times in my life, and how much emotionally stronger I was than other people I knew. I thought mentally ill people were eccentric. Although I behaved oddly by looking for food and sending money abroad that I should have kept for myself, my personality was not eccentric. I believe that my closest friends never saw me that way, even when I was severely ill.

At the hospital, after a few days, the doctors determined I was still psychotic. By observing my behavior, they knew I was hearing voices. Initially, I refused to take a medication that had been prescribed for me. Doctors told me that if I did not take the medication, they would inject it into me without my consent. I chose to begin the oral form of the drug. Unable to recognize I was ill, I demanded a court date to try to secure my release from the ward. I met with a patients' rights representative who listened to me talk about returning "home." I just wanted to be spending my days in the rose garden again.

§

    I began taking Risperdal a few days after arriving at the hospital. After I began taking it, a few important things happened. My painful tactile hallucinations were greatly reduced. Suffering from hallucinations of being jabbed in the back along my spine was one of the most horrible experiences of my life. But though Risperdal helped significantly, it did not eliminate the pain. Rather than see that my pain was lessened, I thought only of pain I still had, and the drug was disappointing to me.

    On Risperdal, almost miraculously, the voices no longer controlled my behavior. I no longer walked right or left at their command, shouted obscenities out loud, or hit myself when they told me to. When I was later released from the hospital, I did not want to look for leftover food in public places where people were around. I was in control of myself again.

    But the voices were not gone. I continued to hear them in the backdrop of my mind, loudly yelling and swearing at me all the time. They were like a broken record, still telling me I was homeless, and they were louder than they had been when they controlled my behavior. This prevented me from reading well, though I could read better on the medication than without it. I was still in denial that I had been incapable of studying in college for years. I did not recognize that the medication improved my reading.

    In addition to the medication's other benefits, all of my other auditory, visual and olfactory hallucinations were immediately and completely eliminated, even after only a few days. The pain and the voices were so resistant to the medication, whereas the other hallucinations were gone so quickly and completely. Even now, my doctor and I do not know why. The voices and the residual pain continued to bother me greatly. I hardly noticed when other hallucinations dissipated because the voices and pain were so strong.

    After just a few days on the medication, I had a desire to return home and live with my parents. My parents later encouraged me to call and reconnect with my brother and our extended family. Because of the medication, I would be able to live in a home without feeling I was trapped in a videogame, feeling bored, or feeling like I was in jail.

The medication changed my state of mind, but I did not know it was happening. I always believed during my four years of homelessness that I could have returned home to my parents if I wanted. I thought my changed desire to live with my family again was my own choice. I did not realize that the medication had eliminated a psychosis that stopped me from being able to stand living in a regular home. Miraculously, it eliminated that psychosis completely.

While in the psychiatric hospital, I was blind to all of the benefits from the medication. I chose not to share with the doctors that I used to experience auditory and visual hallucinations, was still hearing voices in my mind despite the medication, or that I still felt painful tactile hallucinations. I knew I was still hallucinating, but I believed the doctors could do nothing for me. I saw none of the changes Risperdal had made. I was sure I was right, that antipsychotic medications would never do me any good.

While at the hospital, after I had been in the ward for a few days, I met with a counselor, a friendly young woman. I recognized I might need counseling. I told her a little about Africa and my years as a student at the nearby university. But by the time I met her, I had been on medication for at least a few days, and the drug made me lethargic, exhausted and forgetful. I was disappointed to see that the counselor had little interest in talking with me for more than a few minutes.

§

After I spoke with my parents on the phone at the psychiatric ward, they flew out to see me. They arrived about twenty-four hours after I had been picked up on the morning of March 3rd. I saw my parents for the first time during visiting hours in the psychiatric hospital. They looked older, but healthy. My dad was wearing half glasses, which I never saw him wear before. My mom's hair was still blonde, though my dad's was graying.

My parents brought me new clothes, shoes and ice cream. They strongly urged me to cancel the court date I had demanded to secure my release from the ward and to follow the advice of my doctors instead. Because of them and the clearing of my mind from the medication, I did cancel the court date.

My parents invited me to return with them to Cincinnati, where they had resided for five years. They seemed to genuinely want me to move into their home and live with them again. They told me all about their church and community. The said there was a library within walking distance, along with many restaurants and shops. My mom still loved gardening. Later, when I returned home with them, the spring flowers were just beginning to open.

CHAPTER TWENTY-EIGHT

I found it remarkable that the physicians were able to observe patients and determine whether they were hearing voices. In the hospital, I was sometimes walking repeatedly in and out of rooms, choosing to get something to eat and then throwing it away untouched, and not making sense. When I was acting this way, the doctors knew I was hearing voices. They could often recognize patients were hearing voices after just a few minutes.

Since my medication changed the character of the voices, and they stopped commanding me to do things, my behavior changed. But even though the voices stopped affecting my behavior so much, they were still present in my mind all the time like a radio blasting between channels at a high volume, or a song in my head that had exploded into high volume. When I was growing up, I thought hearing voices was the most bizarre thing that could happen to a person. Because of the stigma, I decided I would never tell anyone at any time I was actually hearing voices. And part of me still did not believe it was happening. Regardless, that March after my behavior changed (although I was still secretly hearing voices), doctors determined that I was stable enough to fly back to the Ohio.

After my release from the psychiatric ward, but prior to flying back to Ohio, I faced the humiliation of a mandatory court appearance. I had missed my court appearance that had been scheduled for December 2006. My parents spoke with a public defender and worked out the details for me to appear in court. I still believed I was never wrong in my time at the university, and that I had not been trespassing. But my parents told me I needed to plead no contest, and I would be released.

The judge ruled I was guilty of disturbing the peace, and that I had already served my time in jail. I told her I was ill and under the care of a physician, and she waived a fee that the public defender told me I would have to pay. Though I hated going to court, it was a relief to make my mandatory court appearance and then to move forward with my life. The judge told me that after eighteen months, I could apply to have my criminal records expunged. My legal file was closed less than two years later.

Without the support of my parents or others, I doubt I ever would have attended court on my own. It would have been difficult to go to court while living on the street since I had no identification, and my clothes were dirty. I rarely was aware of the exact date. I am thankful my parents cared enough to support me and enable me to make my court appearance before I flew with them to Cincinnati.

§

In late March, after the hospital psychiatrists discharged me on Risperdal, I flew back to Ohio with my parents. While I was in the psychiatric hospital, I felt much more tired than usual. I spent many more hours asleep, but I thought that it was because there was little to do at the hospital, and I was bored. After I was on the medication for a couple weeks (right after I returned to my parents' home) I found that the medication was making me sleep four to six more hours every day in addition to my usual seven. Eventually, the medication would make me sleep sixteen to eighteen hours every night.

With time, the excess sleep induced by the medication was nothing compared to a side effect called anhedonia, an inability to experience pleasure, where one quickly turns away from beautiful sights, smells or good feelings. This side effect caused me to turn away from pleasure in the same way a person would pull back from an overwhelmingly poignant, horrible smell or pain.

After moving to Cincinnati, I visited relatives who lived in a beautiful forested area of Wisconsin. I looked up at the clear blue sky one afternoon in the forest, and at that moment, something inside of me pulled away from the wonderful feeling. It was like I had stepped on a thorn at the same moment I looked at the sky. The experience was truly horrible, and impossible to forget.

During my trip to Wisconsin, I saw my brother for the first time in about five years. He noticed I was drugged, appeared to be in pain, and was not myself. He cared about me, but we were not really able to talk. I wanted to ask him about his life and work, but I felt too miserable.

§

For me, anhedonia, the inability to experience pleasure, took a few weeks to set in, and I first experienced it about a week after returning to Ohio, and later in Wisconsin. Some patients with Parkison's Disease experience the same anhedonia that I did as a side effect of my medication. I began to feel it every day.

On Risperdal, I became constantly clumsy, though I never had been before. I experienced another side effect called akathisia where I was restless and uncomfortable every minute I was awake, and my arms and legs began to feel tense and heavy. My akathisia never improved while I was on Risperdal, and it made me continually restless every minute. I would walk for miles at a time to try to fight the akathisia, but no amount of walking took the restlessness away. It was always with me, and it was horrible.

The worst side effect I experienced on Risperdal was my severe continuing and worsening anhedonia. Because of this strong and complete pulling away, I could never feel any pleasure at any time. I used to watch carefree dogs and cats run around, happy. I could not experience their carefree, pleasurable feelings because of my medication.

Taking my medication was the opposite of taking an aspirin. Rather than lessening pain, it gave me something worse. I became even more clumsy and dropped things. I gained ten pounds. My mind was becoming more and more oblivious to my surroundings, and I felt like a vegetable in constant pain. For me, life on a "therapeutic dose" of Risperdal was a horrible life.

In addition to all the side effects I had to endure on the medication, the voices were still screaming at me constantly, and they were noticeably louder than they were when they controlled my behavior. I heard the "savior" in my mind telling me he was not interested in me anymore because I was on medication. The painful hallucinations were still not gone. My need for sleep got even worse, and I slept from eight P.M. until noon most days, and still felt sleep-deprived.

As the side effects of Risperdal set in, I imagined I would rather be on chemotherapy or even die than continue to experience the side effects. All I wanted was to be in the state I was in before I began taking it. I associated my homelessness with having good physical health, and I wished I could be homeless again. Though I was mentally ill while I was living at the church, I had felt resilient and energized every day there.

While on medication, I never told anyone how badly I wanted to be homeless again. I knew that it would sound crazy, and that saying it would be hurtful to my parents, who had done everything in their power to make me happy in their home.

On Risperdal, suffering, the desire to stop the medication was with me every hour. Many people have success on Risperdal, and there are some patients who even ask for the medication. For me, it was a nightmare.

§

When I returned to my parents' home, I came to believe that the side effects of Risperdal would make me sick enough to have to return to the psychiatric ward. I remembered who I used to be. I knew that I had no trouble staying home while I was growing up. I did not remember how unhappy and out of focus I had been visiting home after I began studying at the university. I believed that I was emotionally strong, and that if I made the choice to stay home and act as I did in high school, I could do it. I faintly heard the "savior" in my mind demanding that I discontinue medication, and I thought he was right.

In April 2007, about a week after I moved to Cincinnati, I stopped taking Risperdal without telling anyone. I felt greatly relieved and ready to begin enjoying my parents' home. Unfortunately, my decision to go off medication would soon prove to be the wrong one.

CHAPTER TWENTY-NINE

A few days after I stopped Risperdal, I went to a family doctor to get a routine checkup, and he wrote a prescription for more Risperdal. I told him I believed I did not need the medication. He agreed with me that I might not need it, but he said that I should speak with a professional counselor about my illness. I rejected his advice, believing that I needed to talk to no one. During the next two weeks after I discontinued the drug, my intense, daily medication-induced suffering started to disappear.

After a few days off medication, I again saw life as a videogame in which I was trapped. It was hard to deal with living in a home again. After about a week, I badly wanted to leave my parents' home to become homeless. For two weeks after discontinuing Risperdal, I became psychotic in other ways. I was turning into a different person again, the street person.

I did not want to file for medical benefits in Ohio, though my parents and doctors told me I was eligible and should apply immediately. I had signed paperwork to receive medical benefits while I was in the psychiatric hospital out west. The paperwork for medical benefits in Ohio was easy, and benefits would immediately cover the cost of my medication, which was several hundred dollars per month. Off medication, asking for government aid felt humiliating to me. I felt like society was a pyramid, and that if I were living on the government, I would be at the very bottom. In my psychosis, I acutely felt that accepting any government benefits would mean I was a failure.

When I returned to Ohio, an old friend mailed me one of my old violins she had taken and stored for me for nearly five years. I was practicing my old violin again one day at my parents' church when the voices reappeared. They reminded me of a story in the Bible where a woman spilled a bottle of perfume in front of Jesus to honor him. They demanded that in the same way the woman smashed the bottle of perfume, I had to honor God by smashing my violin. They were making no sense. Without medication, I could not choose to go against the voices. At that moment, the voices told me to smash my violin, and I smashed it on the floor.

Seeing my violin in broken pieces was one of the most painful moments of my life. The violin was a gift from my parents when I was thirteen, and it held so many special memories for me. It was one of my favorite possessions I have ever owned, one of my treasures. I was devastated.

Even after my violin was ruined, the voices continued controlling me. I started yelling that I wanted to return out west. I felt I was in jail by living in Cincinnati, just as much as I had been in jail in 2006. In some ways, going off medication while living with my parents felt worse than my second experience being incarcerated in 2006. At least in jail, I was comforted by the isolation. That April of 2007, completely controlled by the voices, I could not stand to be a normal part of a community or to live in a home.

My dad heard me yelling out from his office at the church. When he came, I had a feeling that he cared about me. A group of EMTs and police arrived moments after I broke my violin, though I did not know who called them. Minutes later, my mom appeared on the scene. I was surprised to see her. I told myself over and over again that she was there by chance and not because she was called as a result of my behavior. She talked with some police officers or EMTs in another room. Years later, I learned that when she arrived, she spoke with me at length about my need to go back to the hospital, but I have no memory of our conversation. I remember speaking to her only after I arrived at the hospital.

An officer told me that I had to go to the psychiatric hospital. The officers said that if I would not comply, I would be handcuffed. I complied and went with them.

§

The day I broke my violin, it had been about three weeks since I stopped taking Risperdal. After I was admitted to a psychiatric ward, I met with a physician. Over the years, when I was not psychotic, I often appeared self-controlled and healthy. I talked with the psychiatrist very briefly, and he told me I would be out soon, after a day or two. I did not explain to the doctor that I had been prescribed Risperdal and stopped taking it. Sometimes it seemed I was able to fool members of the hospital staff. It took several weeks for the medication to become eliminated from my blood, so it was still working a little. I was not yet screaming back at the voices all the time or shouting profanity.

After I met with the doctor, my mom met with him. She explained that I was flagrantly psychotic, though I did not always appear to be. After she narrated to him my long psychiatric history, the doctors decided to keep me at the hospital for several days, though they had told me that I would be out after a day or two. I am sure I would have had to return to the hospital again several days or weeks later if they had not kept me there for treatment. I do not know how much damage I might have done if I had been free and off medication for several more days.

The hospital required that I apply for both medical benefits and social security income. I had no choice. Before I left the hospital, a representative sat with me and helped me fill out the more complicated paperwork necessary to apply for social security income. I could not tolerate filling out the paperwork for aid while I was psychotic. But when I was on medication, it made sense.

At the hospital, I started Risperdal again and was sent home. From March to June 2007 I was suffering day to day on Risperdal, and there was not a single day when I had relief. But the drug was working. I was able to live safely in my parents' home without feeling like it was a crowded jail cell.

§

When I returned to the Midwest in 2007, I met a woman with esophageal cancer. I have often wondered whether I would prefer to be in the position of this woman or continue taking Risperdal. I cannot imagine how bad my hallucinations may have become without any medication. It is better for people with schizophrenia to take medications that are available like Risperdal than to have no relief from their hallucinations. Though I hated to take Risperdal, I would rather take it than nothing.

I was only on Risperdal for a few months, until midsummer of 2007, when I met my new Ohio outpatient psychiatrist. This was the lowest point of my life. I badly wished every day that I could be homeless again. The medication made me feel so awful that my homelessness looked exciting and comfortable in comparison.

That summer, my new outpatient psychiatrist took me off Risperdal and put me on Invega, a drug that had recently come out. The new medication was known for not causing the anhedonia and akathisia I experienced on Risperdal. A few weeks after switching to the new medication, my experience of the terrible side effects of pulling away from pleasure began to subside. My extreme restlessness and the tension and heaviness in my limbs also began to disappear. I stopped dropping things easily.

I suffered greatly on Risperdal. I still had a great will to live, and was not suicidal, but I wished most days I could somehow escape from my life of severe pain. Anhedonia and other horrible side effects of medications like Risperdal are sometimes permanent in patients, even after the medication is discontinued. But for me, after only a few weeks, I became mostly free of many of the side effects.

Unfortunately, I found that Invega greatly affected my personality. It made me unable to respond to people quickly. I was extremely sedated by the medication. On both Risperdal and Invega, I acted like a nervous child. Since my natural personality is open and outgoing, I was no longer myself. Though the personality changes were similar on both Risperdal and Invega, I was suffering so much on Risperdal that I did not really notice the changes in myself. On both medications, friends I still had in Cincinnati (from 2001 when I spent Christmas there) became uninterested in me because of how I changed. Both medications, Risperdal and Invega, put me in a sort of mental "fog" where I could not easily remember things, respond quickly or act like myself in social settings.

Fortunately, from spring 2007 onward, several kind people from my parents' church occasionally offered to take me shopping, out to lunch, and downtown to the concert hall. A friend invited me to visit her on her university campus where I was allowed to audit a couple of her classes. These people were extremely compassionate and overlooked my drugged appearance.

§

Prior to beginning antipsychotic medications, I was thin, and had never gained significant weight at any time in my whole life. On both medications, I did everything in my power to not gain weight, but

Risperdal made me gain ten pounds, and Invega made me gain another ten pounds. In the beginning, after I ate a normal meal, I would say to myself "I will not eat" over and over again to stop eating. I sat down on a couch in my parents' home, determined to not eat more and wait until my cravings went away. But after about twenty minutes of repeatedly saying to myself "I will not eat," and sitting there doing nothing, I would give up. I tried it several times, but I would always begin eating again. I had to eat a lot of extra food just to have the energy to do anything, and my best efforts to not overeat were useless. After I gained twenty pounds on the medications, I began feeling some arthritic pain in my back.

About a year later, when I switched to another medication, fifteen pounds of what I gained would quickly fall off.

In addition to this weight gain, Invega also made me sleep sixteen to eighteen hours a night, and like Risperdal, it made me feel sedated all the time. Taking a shower in the morning was as exhausting as practicing violin for four hours used to be. I had become like a sick and weak elderly person. Yet I was only twenty-five years old.

During my life, most of my strengths have been in music and academics. The voices hated my violin and music as much as they hated for me to read. In 2007, on both medications, the voices were no longer controlling me, and I was able to enjoy music again. I was thankful that I could play the violin a little, though not like when I was in high school. I was extremely careful with the violin a church member gave me in late spring of 2007.

Besides playing the violin, all I wanted was to read and study, so that I might finally be myself. Though Invega was an improvement over Risperdal, I was a vegetable on both medications. Though I could play the violin a little and read some, I could not study.

While on Risperdal and then Invega, I stopped making plans for the future and had no goals or dreams. In the past, I always had goals and dreams, even while hearing the voices that began in 2006. At one point, in summer 2007, I tried visiting a professor of molecular biology at the University of Cincinnati to discuss my research. He seemed interested in me, but I was too sedated and distracted to be able to discuss my research like I used to. Invega was better than

Risperdal, but my whole future depended on finding a medication that really worked, one that could give me back my life. It was not until I found a medication that really worked that I would again begin to have goals, hopes and dreams, such as studying molecular biology again.

CHAPTER THIRTY

One day in summer 2007, right after I had switched to Invega, I was speaking with my dad, and he expressed his concern about me. He wanted to understand why I could not study anymore. I finally gave up, and I told my parents I was hearing voices despite the medication. It was the first time I admitted to anyone that I was hearing voices, or that I had ever heard voices. The voices were under control on Risperdal and Invega, but they had begun a year and a half prior (in January of 2006) and they were still lingering in my mind.

With encouragement from my parents, I took the step of speaking to my psychiatrist about the voices. I explained that while they were not controlling me anymore, they were in my mind, and loud, and that they were with me almost every minute. After I spoke with the psychiatrist about my "residual voices," which I found they were called, the psychiatrist put me on and off various medications. This included Abilify and Geodon from fall 2007 until February 2008.

Abilify and Geodon allowed me to stay in touch with reality, and I no longer felt like I was trapped in a video game. I was still able to have healthy relationships with my mom and dad and a few friends, and able to live in my parents' home without feeling like I was trapped there.

When I switched from Invega to Abilfy and Geodon, my dream of feeling like myself again was coming true. The drugs had remarkably few side effects. I slept far less, and was less sedated and more alert. But the new medications did not counter the voices in my mind. They were still vivid as any dream or as a song in my head that exploded in volume. The voices began yelling even louder, and they began to control me again. It seemed Invega did better at countering the voices than the other medications I tried. I was devastated that the medications with so few side effects did not eliminate the voices.

In February 2008, a year after I moved to Cincinnati, Abilify and Geodon were not working. Weeks after I stopped taking Invega, there were annoying sounds that reappeared in my mind that I had not heard since March 2007. My psychiatrist was not available for weeks at a time. My parents and I tried going to the Psychiatric Emergency Services to get my medication changed, but the physicians there were generally not helpful. They told us we should wait until my appointment with my outpatient psychiatrist. We tried going again and again, hoping each time for a different mental health professional who might be concerned about me and make a significant adjustment in my medications to relieve my suffering.

One night, the noises in my mind made me scream as though I had suffered severe pain, almost as a reflex. My mom and I went to the emergency room again, and a staff member informed us that they could not help me sufficiently unless I was admitted to the hospital again. I voluntarily admitted myself to the psychiatric ward, desperate to try other medications.

§

At the psychiatric ward, a nurse told me that a medication I had not yet tried would definitely work to alleviate my voices as it had worked for millions of others. It was called Zyprexa. But she also told me that I might gain fifty or possibly even a hundred pounds, "blowing up like a balloon." A nurse warned me that a single dose of the medication might permanently make me a diabetic. But I had to try it. My life was at stake.

When I began Zyprexa at the hospital, I was surprised that it did not make me gain weight. It did not make my limbs tense and heavy. But for as much as the medication had few side effects, it did not eliminate the voices. I almost felt like I was taking a placebo.

I was in the hospital for several days. Eventually, I realized that Invega had been better. Though it was a horrible drug for me, and even like a nightmare, Invega allowed me to live outside the psychiatric hospital. After several days in the ward with nothing else working, I asked for Invega so that I could go home. The hospital psychiatrist sent me home on the same dosage of Invega I took before. It was frustrating to leave just where I had started.

§

Before leaving the psychiatric ward, my psychiatrist spoke with me about a medication called Clozaril, which he said was a "gold-standard" medication. The doctor said it was only prescribed to patients who were not responsive to any of the other antipsychotic medications, or who experienced horrible side effects on other medications.

Of all the drugs on the American market, Clozaril was considered the worst for weight gain. But apart from this weight gain, sedating patients, and causing patients to sleep longer, the medication was known to generally have no side effects. The problem with the medication was that a few patients had died from taking it when it was used without close monitoring. Due to potential side effects, patients on the medication were required to have weekly blood tests for a year, and then monthly blood tests. My psychiatrist told me that many patients who had spent years in psychiatric hospitals recovered on Clozaril and went home.

The doctors determined I was stable on Invega and could return to live with my parents. They arranged to have my new outpatient psychiatrist prescribe me a low dose of Clozaril, which would be added to my Invega. I saw my new outpatient psychiatrist a week after I left the hospital.

In February 2008, I left the psychiatric ward for the third and last time.

§

The following week, I met with a mental health professional who was highly recommended by the hospital physicians. When I met him, he told me that I would never be able to return to college, or at least not for many years. He thought there was no possibility that I would make a significant recovery. He spoke to me slowly as though I were a child. The professional suggested I attend a day program where many of the participants were people who had abused drugs, which made me feel uncomfortable. Participating in a day program indefinitely was not what I envisioned for my life. What I wanted most was to return to college. But if college were not possible, I wanted to spend my time reading, playing my violin, and enjoying activities with people who were *not* mentally ill. The program did not seem to be a good fit, and I decided not to participate in it. But even if I had wanted to, it would have been impossible since I was sleeping sixteen to eighteen hours a day.

When I finally met my new outpatient psychiatrist, he initially decided to raise my dose of Zyprexa instead of trying Clozaril, but it did not work.

My new psychiatrist felt that speaking with a counselor would not be helpful to me. He thought my disease was a result of a chemical imbalance in my brain and felt that only medications could alleviate my suffering. I had no childhood trauma or other trauma apart from what I encountered overseas. Months after I began my first antipsychotic medication, I was able to deal with the poverty I had seen overseas and finally grieve. In 2007, when I first returned to Cincinnati, I met with a counselor, but did not feel she was helpful. I never benefitted from counseling.

§

My parents wanted me to have a life beyond support groups and day programs. They hoped that someday I could work a job, and encouraged me to not give up. They never gave up hope that I might return to study at a university again. We all wanted another opinion, and my parents were persistent.

While I was in the hospital, some of the doctors spoke about my case with a university professor who was a well-known specialist in schizophrenia. They explained that I was intelligent, and was searching for a medication that might enable me to return to the university. The university professor spoke with my mom, and he agreed to consult with my doctor. Together, the doctors put me on Clozaril. I consented to have the required weekly blood tests. Just when I thought all hope was lost, I began the medication.

§

Since Clozaril was infamous for causing severe weight gain, I anticipated gaining twenty or thirty pounds during my first few weeks on the medication. But over the first few weeks, I was less hungry, and I began losing weight. Within a couple of months, I lost fifteen pounds. My many hours of sleeping were reduced. I went from sixteen or eighteen hours a night to twelve.

By April 2008, several weeks later, my long-awaited miracle finally occurred, and the voices were quieter. I was becoming free of the screaming chorus of children's voices and other characters that lived in my mind for two and a half years. They had been with me nearly every minute I was awake.

I had felt for years that only a miracle could take the mental fog away. It was beginning to clear on Clozaril, and after a few more weeks, I saw significant improvement. My mind became more like it was in 2001 or 2002, before I went to Boston, where I flew hoping to meet an imaginary "savior" who never arrived to meet me at the airport. I did not have side effects such as restlessness, inability to experience pleasure, or the need to overeat. I was no longer childlike, sedated and shy. It truly was a miracle.

It was possible for me to go out into the community again and begin making friends. I went to social events with confidence, met new friends and spent time with them. I almost felt like my old self again, the way I felt during high school and during my first semester at the university.

For the first time since 2006, I began to read books. I started with easy books, like reading the *Chronicles of Narnia* again and the *Anne of Green Gables* series. I soon progressed to reading history and philosophy books. I remembered what I read and was regaining my ability to study.

After a year on Clozaril, the voices were virtually gone. I was healthy and thin again. I had recovered.

CHAPTER THIRTY-ONE

With encouragement from my parents, I prepared to continue my university education. I was accepted at the University of Cincinnati and transferred my credits there. I found an apartment I loved near campus. A year and a half after I began Clozaril, my parents helped me move, and I enrolled at the university.

I started school slowly in fall of 2009. I took just one class, genetics, and earned an A. With bolstered confidence, I took neurobiology and microbiology the next quarter. I realized I was capable of finishing my bachelor's degree in molecular biology. Returning to university study was one of the happiest times of my life. I thought going back to school would never be possible. I loved being in school again and was grateful for it every day.

During Christmas of 2009, I enjoyed spending time with family. I helped decorate the tree, went shopping with my mom, and joined my family for our annual Christmas dinner. I was happy, and no longer restless.

I had only seen my brother once after returning to the Midwest. Our meeting in Wisconsin had been brief, and we could not converse much because I was highly medicated and suffering. My brother now lived out west and did not visit often. I had spoken frequently with him over the phone since I moved to Cincinnati. That Christmas, I was well enough to enjoy spending time with him in person. We talked about his job, his interests and his life out west, as well as my new classes. My family was finally together again, and happy.

As I continued to study at the university, I enjoyed classes as I always had before I became ill. The only problem was my medication-induced exhaustion, which caused me to continue sleeping about twelve hours every night. I was still tired most days as though I had not slept enough. Because I slept so much, I could only attend the university part-time. I wished I could reduce my time asleep to seven hours each night. I tried exercising and changing my diet, but saw no effect. I missed my high school years when I was taking a full-time course load, always getting straight A's, and practicing violin for hours every day. Sometimes I missed my first years at the university out west. I was able to work in the laboratory most nights past midnight. I could take many difficult classes at the same time and score high grades.

The summer after my first year at the University of Cincinnati, I did research with a professor at the university medical school. I read widely on my project and enjoyed being in a laboratory again, but unlike previous years, laboratory work was exhausting for me.

In August 2010, my doctor put me on a second medication called Provigil (I later switched to Nuvigil). The medication made me more alert, and it enabled me to study or work for several more hours every week. I was able to take more credit hours at the university, though I still could not attend college full-time. The medication gave me the energy to give a good presentation of my summer research in August 2010. On Provigil, I finally had the energy to review some of the Chinese and Hebrew I used to study.

In fall 2010, I continued school. I took physics and a philosophy course and got A's in both. I found myself able to study or work twenty or twenty-five hours a week, though it may be sixty hours for others. I was able to learn new Chinese vocabulary on my own.

I graduated with my molecular biology degree in December 2011, two years after enrolling at the university. My university GPA was 3.84. I was chosen to be one of eight marshals in my college graduation ceremony. Marshals wore a special red cap and gown which stood out against the traditional black cap and gown. Walking with the other seven marshals, I led the graduating class into the auditorium to receive their degrees. My parents, brother, some close friends, and my psychiatrist attended my graduation. It was one of the best days of my life, but I think my doctor was even happier about my graduation than I was. I think he saw it as a major victory and milestone rarely achieved in his career. I will never forget that day.

Shortly after, I took the Graduate Record Examination (GRE) and received a high score.

§

After taking the GRE, I began the arduous task of writing this book, my memoir. I do not consider myself healed from schizophrenia, but I am fully recovered. I want to be a spokesperson for people desperately impaired by psychoses, and bring the good news that, today, mentally ill people can have happy and productive lives. I hope that, someday, psychiatric patients will be treated with compassion like people with infections, cancer patients and people with all other diseases of the body.

Above all, I hope that people who read my memoir will better understand mentally ill homeless people. America's jails are full of many individuals who are mentally ill like I was. They need and deserve psychiatric treatment, and a second chance at life.

AFTERWORD

Today, after recovering from my illness, I find myself living a rewarding life. My life is full of wonderful relationships. I am close friends again with my parents and extended family. I attend a church and social gatherings through the University of Cincinnati. I have dated young men, and greatly enjoyed these relationships. I play violin often for gatherings. Every Easter weekend, I look forward to joining a small orchestra that performs excerpts from Handel's Messiah. I love playing my violin for services at Christmastime.

I am delighted to meet international students at the university. Studying other languages and cultures continues to be one of the highlights of my life. I have had more than one Chinese speaker laugh at me as I speak their language, and call me "hao wan," which means "lots of fun." The vitality and quick wit of my many international friends keeps my life interesting.

When I attended the University of Cincinnati from 2009 until my graduation in 2011, I was thankful every day to be studying molecular biology, particularly courses which included information about mental illnesses. Today, I am determined to study and better understand schizophrenia and other mental illnesses. Physicians at the University of Cincinnati welcome me to attend a "grand rounds" seminar every week within the medical school, and I attend other seminars and gatherings where researchers engage in discussions on recent developments in psychiatry. Doctors are developing brain scans that will show a patient has mental illness before symptoms appear. It seems that in the future, doctors will be able to treat patients before the onset of mental illnesses. Doctors wonder if, someday, mental illness may become as treatable as diabetes. The developments in the field are amazing.

For the past two years, since I graduated from the University of Cincinnati, a combination of writing this memoir, learning about mental illness, and speaking to groups of doctors and mental health professionals about my life, on a confidential basis, has become my multifaceted "job." I still cannot work full-time because I am tired every day due to my medication, and because the medication continues to make me sleep twelve hours a night. As a speaker, I have found audiences are eager to hear my story and are very encouraging to me, which is one of the reasons I was encouraged by my psychiatrist to write this memoir. At the same time, almost none of my friends know my medical history. It has been impossible to share with my friends that I have spent most of my time these last two years writing down my life story. A professor recommended I tell friends I am doing a "research project in psychiatry" until the time when this memoir is published.

Professionally, when I interact with university psychiatrists, there are only a very few who know about my past symptoms and recovery. But occasionally, I run into physicians who knew me when I was in the hospital in 2008 for ten days. Some of these doctors are shocked when they realize that I am the same person they treated. Most of them saw the seriousness of my illness and assumed that a full recovery, like I have made, would never be possible.

In one of my social gatherings at the University of Cincinnati, there is a homeless person who regularly comes to a student facility, where he is not allowed to be. Staff members have told him many times not to enter the facility, and have filed a trespassing order to keep him away. Sometimes, I see other homeless people on the streets of Cincinnati holding signs or sleeping on the concrete. Because I lived as a homeless person for four years, I know how these people feel. Every day, I look forward to another time in my life when I can be honest with people about my life, and how ill I really was, and homeless, just like the homeless people I see near the campus. Because I have not been able to share my illness and recovery with others, I often feel like I am living under a shadow. By writing this book, I hope to come out of the shadow. Until I do, I doubt I can ever experience fulfilling relationships and truly find happiness.

I have many hopes for the future. I hope to get married someday, and also to continue my studies, either through formal or informal education. But above all, I hope that by writing this book under my real name, I can step out of the shadow. I am excited to see what the future holds.

ACKNOWLEDGEMENTS

I offer my deepest thanks to Dr. Henry Nasrallah, whose dedicated care has been foundational in my full recovery from schizophrenia. He has been not only a devoted physician, but a mentor and a guide. His compassionate skill and belief in my potential gave me the courage and confidence to keep setting my goals higher and higher. I believe he will never cease to challenge me to accomplish things that once looked impossible.

I am especially indebted to both of my parents who loved me through a very difficult chapter of my life and committed themselves to my recovery, that I might have a second chance. Without them, I doubt I would ever have finished college. I cherish their loving support and friendship. I am also grateful to them for their help editing this manuscript and for providing helpful suggestions.

I am grateful to my advisor Dr. Matthew Sauer for his professional support and guidance while I was a student at the University of Cincinnati, and for his support and insight regarding the development and arrangement of this manuscript.

I thank my editor, Gretchen Dietz, whose dedicated work has been invaluable. I appreciate her patience and tenacity through many revisions.

I thank Alex Friedman for editing and formatting my manuscript. I thank Theresa Ware for her photography, and graphic artist Ryan Martin for contributing to the design of the book.

ABOUT THE AUTHOR

Bethany Yeiser holds a bachelor's degree in molecular biology with honors from the University of Cincinnati. Prior to becoming homeless, she published three articles in biochemistry, including a first-authored article in *Proceedings of the National Academy of Sciences*. In 2000, she presented a first-authored poster at the Interscience Conference on Antimicrobial Agents and Chemotherapy. She began full-time college at age fifteen and transferred to a well-known university on the West Coast at seventeen.

Bethany spent three months living and volunteering in the slums of Nairobi, Kenya and in Lagos, Nigeria during the summer of 2002. On her return, in October, 2002, she incorporated a small nonprofit organization to channel money into indigenous African medical missions. It received tax-exempt status in March 2003, and raised several thousand dollars to build a new clinic in Nairobi, Kenya in August of 2003.

Bethany is an accomplished violinist. She has performed in orchestras, worked for recording studios, and taught violin. Bethany was diagnosed with schizophrenia in 2007 after spending four years as a homeless person, including one year spent with only one change of clothes, and living in a churchyard. Today, she is an invited speaker at numerous conferences for physicians and health care providers who seek to learn more about schizophrenia. Bethany has studied ancient Hebrew and Mandarin Chinese.

Mind Estranged is her first book.

FURTHER READING

Flight from Reason:
A Mother's Story of Schizophrenia, Recovery and Hope
A memoir by Karen S. Yeiser

Flight from Reason is the companion book to *Mind Estranged: My Journey from Schizophrenia and Homelessness to Recovery.* While *Mind Estranged* is Bethany's story written from Bethany's perspective, *Flight from Reason* chronicles the agony a loving parent suffers by losing a child to schizophrenia.

Seen through Karen's eyes, and with raw honesty, she brings the reader directly into her own world of confusion and heartbreak. During a five year estrangement, Bethany fled from family and friends while schizophrenia twisted her sense of reality.

Karen helplessly watched her kind and gifted daughter drop out of college, follow an obsession to travel alone into remote parts of the world, and eventually land homeless on the streets of a big city. At times Karen did not know if Bethany was dead or alive.

Flight from Reason carries the reader alongside the depths of illness and will broaden your understanding of how untreated mental illness can devastate families. Against all odds Bethany made a surprising and complete recovery.

Flight from Reason parallels the timeline of *Mind Estranged.* It will encourage and inspire people with mental illness as well as families who love them.

Made in the USA
Columbia, SC
13 January 2021